Manual of
CLINICAL PROCEDURES
IN THE DOG AND CAT

Steven E. Crow, DVM

College of Veterinary Medicine
Michigan State University
East Lansing, Michigan

Sally O. Walshaw, MA, VMD

Veterinary Technology Program
Michigan State University
East Lansing, Michigan

Illustrated by **Cynthia Bronson Morton**

J. B. Lippincott Company
Philadelphia
London   Mexico City   New York
St. Louis   São Paulo   Sydney

Manual of

CLINICAL PROCEDURES IN THE DOG AND CAT

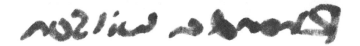

Sponsoring Editor: Delois Patterson
Manuscript Editor: Mary K. Smith
Indexer: Ellen Murray
Art Director: Tracy Baldwin
Design Coordinator: Anne O'Donnell
Designer: Katharine Nichols
Production Manager: Kathleen P. Dunn
Production Editor: Carol A. Florence
Compositor: Circle Graphics
Printer/Binder: R. R. Donnelley & Sons Co.

6   5

Library of Congress Cataloging-in-Publication Data

Crow, Steven E.
  Manual of clinical procedures in the dog and cat.

  Bibliography: p.
  Includes index.
  1. Dogs—Diseases.   2. Cats—Diseases.
3. Veterinary clinical pathology.   I. Walshaw,
Sally O.   II. Title.
SF991.C76 1987   636.7'089   86-10380
ISBN 0-397-50595-7

The authors and publisher have exerted every effort to ensure that drug selection and dosage set forth in this text are in accord with current recommendations and practice at the time of publication. However, in view of ongoing research, changes in government regulations, and the constant flow of information relating to drug therapy and drug reactions, the reader is urged to check the package insert for each drug for any change in indications and dosage and for added warnings and precautions. This is particularly important when the recommended agent is a new or infrequently employed drug.

PREFACE

As instructors of veterinary students and veterinary technology students, we are acutely aware of the deficiencies in clinical training that result from compressed and crowded professional curricula. Many students in veterinary colleges and veterinary technician training programs may never see or perform some very common and important clinical procedures. A consequence of this omission in training is that graduate veterinary technicians and veterinarians are not fully aware of the proper applications and techniques of many in-office procedures. One of our purposes in offering this *Manual of Clinical Procedures in the Dog and Cat* is to encourage more frequent and more correct use of these diagnostic and therapeutic procedures in veterinary practice.

The *Manual* is intended as a textbook for veterinary technology and veterinary students, as well as a useful clinical tool for veterinarians and veterinary technicians in small animal practice or laboratory animal care facilities. Because the text is organized by procedure, and each procedure is described in detail using a step-by-step approach, it can and should be used as a clinical handbook in addition to being a teaching instrument. Features that should make this manual most useful are the rationale/amplification segments, which answer the reader's how and why questions, and the illustrations, which show exactly how to physically manage the patient, equipment, and assistants.

The scope of the *Manual* is limited to procedures that can be completed in most modern veterinary facilities and that require only modest surgical skills. No expensive or complicated equipment is required for any of these techniques, thus they can be cost-effective even in small practices. We have selected procedures that often are needed in everyday practice but either are underused or misused.

It is our hope that the *Manual* will help technicians and veterinarians to make better use of these valuable clinical techniques.

We recommend that the reader use the *Manual* in the following ways:

1. When first learning a procedure, the entire chapter or segment should be studied including purposes, indications, contraindications, possible complications, equipment needed, restraint and positioning, and preparations. This background is essential if proper application of each procedure is to be achieved.
2. Careful attention to comments in the rationale/amplification sections will help the operator to avoid common errors of omission or commission.
3. For subsequent cases, the reader may use the technical action guidelines in a cookbook fashion. Periodic review of other sections of the procedure/description is recommended, however.
4. Careful attention should be paid to Notes that appear throughout the *Manual.*
5. To ensure proper positioning of needles, catheters, and hands, the reader must attempt to duplicate the orientation shown in the line drawings.

If these guidelines are followed, we are confident that the user of the *Manual* can become proficient in a wide variety of diagnostic and therapeutic techniques.

While we try to instruct veterinarians and veterinary technicians in the "how to" of clinical procedures, we hope our equally important message of "whether to" also is understood by the reader. As animal advocates, we have carefully scrutinized each of the procedures with respect to the degree or risk of pain and injury versus expected benefits. We implore our readers to respect the feelings and rights of animals (and their owners) in all aspects of their professional activities.

Steven E. Crow, DVM
Sally O. Walshaw, MA, VMD

"Primum non nocere (first of all do no harm)"

—*Hippocrates*

ACKNOWLEDGMENTS

The authors would like to express their gratitude to the following individuals for their helpful comments during the preparation of this text.

Lorel K. Anderson, DVM
Benjamin H. Colmery, DVM
A. Thomas Evans, DVM
Cheri A. Johnson, DVM
Richard J. Indrieri, DVM
Graham T. Lewis, DVM
Alice Parr, LVT
Richard Walshaw, BVMS
Gail C. Wolz, LVT

CONTENTS

Part 1

ROUTINE CLINICAL PROCEDURES

The procedures described in this section are those commonly performed in small animal practices or laboratory animal facilities. Members of busy veterinary practices are likely to employ these techniques one or more times daily. Proficiency in these procedures will allow veterinarians and technicians to perform their duties more efficiently.

Many readers will have considerable experience with these routine procedures; however, attention to indications, contraindications, and preparations should help even the most experienced clinician to select and apply these techniques more appropriately.

Experience enables you to recognize a mistake when you make it again.

FRANKLIN P. JONES

Chapter 1

RESTRAINT OF DOGS AND CATS

Don't be impatient with your patients.

CARL OSBORNE

Restraint is the restriction of an animal's activity by verbal, physical, or pharmacologic means so that the animal is prevented from injuring itself or others.

Purposes

1. To facilitate physical examination, including ophthalmic and rectal examinations
2. To administer oral, injectable, and topical materials
3. To apply bandages
4. To perform certain procedures (*e.g.,* urinary catheterization)

Complications

1. Dyspnea
2. Hyperthermia

Equipment Needed

- Strips of gauze or cloth, 40 to 60 inches in length, 1 to 2 inches in width, when muzzling is indicated
- Elizabethan collar, when indicated

VERBAL RESTRAINT

Procedure

Technical Action

1. In general, begin with the least severe restraint technique and proceed to more severe methods if necessary.

2. Speak to the dog or cat when approaching it.

3. Use the animal's name.

4. If necessary, speak firmly to the animal.

5. *Assistant:* Stand on opposite side of animal from person performing procedure.

Rationale/Amplification

1. The amount of restraint needed will depend on the environment, the animal's behavior, and the degree of discomfort caused by the procedure.

2. Speaking to the animal initially in a calm, soothing voice helps to prevent startling it. This is especially important if the animal is blind or is looking in another direction.

3. Pet animals are conditioned to respond to their names.

4. Say "no" in a sharp clear tone of voice. Verbal restraint can be a useful adjunct to the physical restraint of pet animals.

5. The intended site for treatment or examination must be easily accessible.

PHYSICAL RESTRAINT WITH DOG IN STANDING POSITION (Fig. 1-1)

Procedure

Technical Action

1. Place one arm under dog's neck so that forearm holds dog's head securely.

2. Place other arm underneath dog's abdomen or thorax.

3. Pull dog close to chest of person performing the restraint.

Rationale/Amplification

1. The dog's head should be positioned so that it is virtually impossible for the dog to bite either the person restraining it or the person performing the procedure.

2. An arm underneath the dog's abdomen will prevent the dog's sitting down during the procedure.

3. The restrainer has more control of the animal's movement if the animal is held close to him or her.

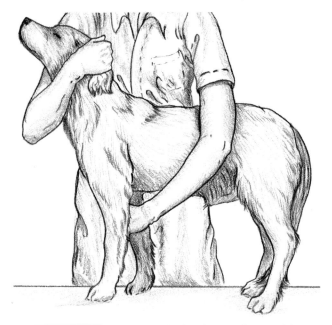

Figure 1-1 Restraint with dog in standing position.

PHYSICAL RESTRAINT WITH DOG SITTING OR IN STERNAL RECUMBENCY (Fig. 1-2)

Procedure

Technical Action

1. Place one arm under dog's neck so that forearm holds dog's head securely.
2. Place other arm around dog's hindquarters.

3. Pull dog close to chest of person doing restraint.

Rationale/Amplification

1. Adequate restraint of the dog's head is important for all procedures.
2. An arm around the dog's hindquarters will prevent the dog from standing up or lying down during the procedure.
3. The restrainer has more control of the animal's movement if the animal is held close to him or her.

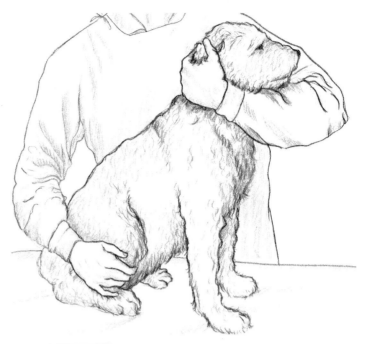

Figure 1-2 Restraint with dog in sitting position.

PHYSICAL RESTRAINT WITH DOG IN LATERAL RECUMBENCY (Fig. 1-3)

Procedure

Technical Action

1. With dog in standing position, reach across dog's back and take hold of both forelegs in one hand and both hindlegs in other hand.

2. Gradually lift dog's legs off table (or floor) and allow its body to slowly slide against your body to a position of lateral recumbency.

3. Use forearm nearer to dog's head to exert pressure on side of head, thus keeping its head immobilized.

Rationale/Amplification

1. If the dog is a giant breed, it will suffice to reach across the dog's back and take hold of the foreleg and the hindleg that are closer to the person doing the restraint.

2. The dog should be shifted from a standing position to lateral recumbency gently and gradually.

3. Adequate restraint of the dog's head is important for all procedures.

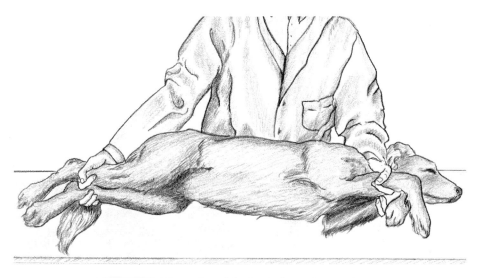

Figure 1-3   Restraint with dog in lateral recumbency.

Technical Action

4. Place index finger of each hand between the two legs being held.

5. Hold legs proximal to carpus and tarsus, if possible.

Rationale/Amplification

4. Placing the index finger between the legs ensures a good grip if the dog tries to move its legs.

5. Holding the animal in this manner provides better control of the legs.

USE OF A MUZZLE IN THE DOG (Fig. 1-4)

Procedure

Technical Action

1. Cut strip of gauze or cloth approximately 50 inches in length for a 40- to 50-lb dog.

2. Before approaching animal, make loop with one half of a square knot so that diameter of loop is about twice the diameter of dog's snout.

Rationale/Amplification

1. Use of sturdy or double-thickness gauze is recommended for large dogs. A poorly made muzzle leads to a false sense of security and the possibility of one's being bitten by the dog.

2. Preparation of the muzzle in advance helps to ensure rapid placement and minimizes the length of time the operator's hands must be near the dog's mouth.

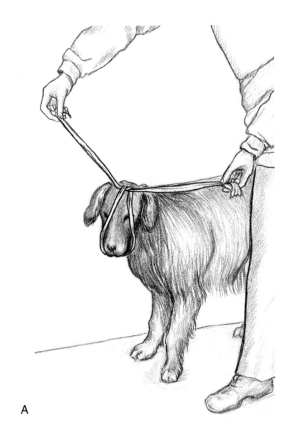

A

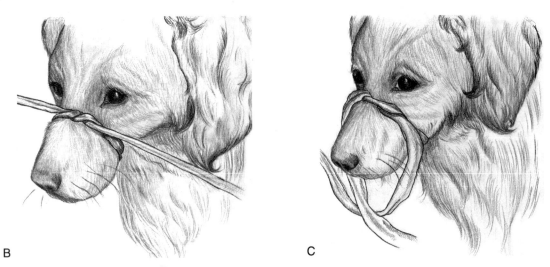

B   C

Figure 1-4 (*A, B, C, D,* and *E*) Applying muzzle to dog.

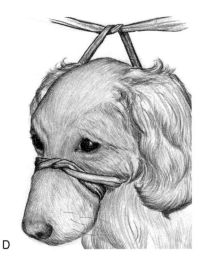

D

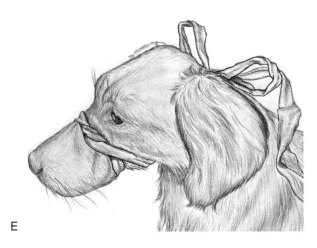

E

Technical Action

3. Slip loop over dog's nose and mouth with the half square knot on dorsal surface of dog's snout (Fig. 1-4*A*), and tighten quickly by pulling on ends (Fig. 1-4*B*).

4. Cross (but do not tie) free ends of muzzle under dog's lower jaw (Fig. 1-4*C*).

5. Bring ends of muzzle up behind dog's ears (Fig. 1-4*D*) and tie in a bow (Fig. 1-4*E*).

6. To remove muzzle quickly from a fractious dog, untie bow and pull on one end of muzzle material.

Rationale/Amplification

3. The hands should be kept as far away from the dog's mouth as possible while the muzzle is applied. Placing a muzzle on a fractious dog requires at least two people: one person holds the leash and distracts the dog while the other applies the muzzle.

4. Each step of this procedure must be done quickly if the animal is fractious. If the ends are crossed but not tied under the mandible, the muzzle can be removed quickly in case of emergency (see No. 6 below).

5. The bow should be placed directly behind the dog's ears and tied tightly. The dog will be able to open its mouth if the muzzle is tied loosely.

6. A muzzle prevents panting and must be used judiciously in heavy-coated animals or in warm environments. A muzzle should be removed immediately if an animal has difficulty breathing or starts to vomit.

USE OF ELIZABETHAN COLLAR (Fig. 1-5)

Procedure

Technical Action

1. Place Elizabethan collar on neck of fractious dog or cat to prevent animal from biting while it is being handled (Fig. 1-5A).

Rationale/Amplification

1. Some advantages of the Elizabethan collar as a restraint device are that the animal can pant with the collar in place; the collar can be left on the animal when it is returned to a hospital kennel, facilitating later removal of the animal for further treatments; the collar is reasonably well tolerated by most animals.

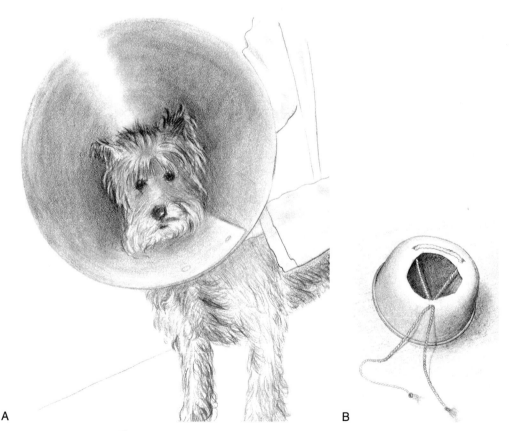

A

B

Figure 1-5 (*A*) Commercial Elizabethan collar on a dog. (*B*) Elizabethan collar constructed from dessert topping container and nylon cord.

Technical Action

2. To ensure that collar will remain on animal, place three holes in container so that a triangular-shaped opening is created for animal's head when cord is passed through the three holes (Fig. 1-5*B*).

Rationale/Amplification

2. Such collars are sturdy, reusable, and easily cleaned. Elizabethan collars for cats and very small dogs can be constructed out of empty dessert topping containers. Collars for dogs can be fashioned from plastic buckets of appropriate sizes.

PHYSICAL RESTRAINT WITH CAT IN LATERAL RECUMBENCY (Fig. 1-6)

Procedure

Technical Action

1. Clip curved end of cat's claws if it must be restrained for lengthy or uncomfortable procedure or if it is fractious (Chap. 11).

2. With cat in standing position, reach across cat's back and take hold of both forelegs in one hand and both hindlegs in other hand.

3. Gradually pull cat's legs off table and allow its back to slide against your body to a position of lateral recumbency.

4. After placing cat in lateral recumbency, use one hand to hold all four legs (Fig. 1-6).

5. Place other hand around cat's head so that palm of hand surrounds dorsal part of cat's head and cat's jaws are held closed by fingers and thumb (Fig. 1-6).

Rationale/Amplification

1. Restraining a cat can be more difficult than restraining a dog for several reasons: a) A cat can move very quickly; b) cats tend to be agile and strong; c) a cat may use its claws as well as its teeth to defend itself; d) a cat is a small animal that could be injured by indiscriminate use of force.

3. The cat should be shifted from a standing position to lateral recumbency gently.

4. If necessary, separate strips of 1-inch-wide adhesive tape can be used to bind together the front legs and the hindlegs respectively.

5. Placing an Elizabethan collar on a fractious cat before beginning the restraint procedure eliminates the necessity of holding the cat's mouth closed with one hand while holding all four legs with the other hand. A cat's small size and

Technical Action

Rationale/Amplification

great agility make immobilization of its head with the restrainer's forearm virtually impossible.

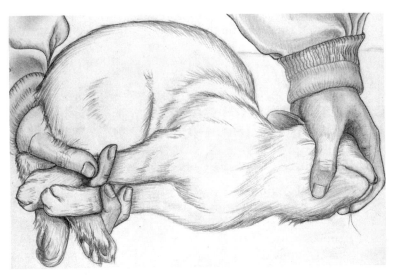

Figure 1-6   Restraint with cat in lateral recumbency.

PHYSICAL RESTRAINT WITH CAT IN STERNAL RECUMBENCY (Fig. 1-7)

Procedure

Technical Action

1. Apply gentle, firm pressure to cat's back to encourage it to assume position of sternal recumbency.
2. Place one forearm against each side of cat's body with cat's head facing away from restrainer.
3. Immobilize cat's head using both hands.

Rationale/Amplification

1. Sternal recumbency is a position to which few cats object.

3. The person doing the procedure can approach from the side or from the cat's rear so as to remain out of reach of the front claws, should the cat attempt to strike.

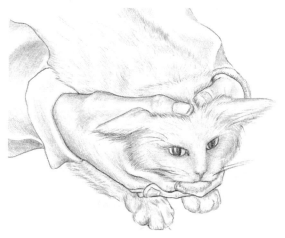

Figure 1-7 Restraint with cat in sternal recumbency.

PHYSICAL RESTRAINT OF MODERATELY FRACTIOUS CAT (Fig. 1-8)

Procedure

Technical Action

1. Close all doors and windows of the room.

2. Take scruff of cat's neck in one hand.

3. With other hand stretch out cat's hindlegs.

4. Hold cat in lateral recumbency or in vertical position.

Rationale/Amplification

1. If the cat gets away from the restrainer, it will not escape from the building.

2. It is important to grasp as much of the loose skin as possible along the anterior portion of the cat's neck, beginning between its ears. Otherwise the cat may be able to turn its head around and bite.

3. Most fractious cats will raise strong vocal protests to this procedure.

4. The necessary procedure should be done quickly. If the restrainer begins to lose control of the cat, he or she should state this to the other person and then let go of the cat with both hands at the same time.

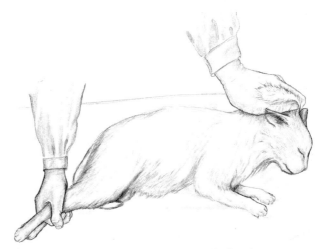

Figure 1-8   Restraint of moderately fractious cat.

Vicious dogs and cats require special restraint techniques, for example, rabies poles and pharmacologic agents. Such procedures carry significant risks for animals and persons involved.

Bibliography

Fowler M: Restraint and Handling of Wild and Domestic Animals. Ames, Iowa State University Press, 1978

Pratt PW (ed): Medical Nursing for Animal Health Technicians. Santa Barbara, American Veterinary Publications, 1985

Wolz G: Personal Communication, 1982

Chapter 2

BLOOD COLLECTION

It is impossible for anyone to begin to learn what he thinks he already knows.

EPICTETUS

ROUTINE VENIPUNCTURE

Routine venipuncture is the placement of a needle into a vein.

Purposes

1. To obtain a sample of venous blood for routine clinical pathology tests, for example, complete blood count (CBC) and serum chemistry determinations
2. To administer medications, fluids, blood, and certain test substances

Complications

1. Minor hemorrhage
2. Subcutaneous hematoma formation
3. Vascular trauma
4. Thrombophlebitis

Equipment Needed

- Cotton
- 70% alcohol or other skin disinfectant
- 3-ml or 10-ml syringe or Vacutainer* holder
- 20- to 22-gauge, 1-inch hypodermic needle

* Becton–Dickinson Co., Rutherford, NJ.

- Blood collection tubes, with or without anticoagulant, depending on laboratory tests to be performed
- Adhesive tape, 1 inch wide

Restraint and Positioning

Routine blood collection in dogs and cats generally requires two persons: one obtains the blood sample while the other restrains the animal. For an uncooperative dog, muzzling may be necessary. An Elizabethan collar is useful for the restraint of an uncooperative cat or brachycephalic dog.

Position for Collection From Jugular Vein

1. Place animal in sternal recumbency on table.
2. With one hand, grasp animal's front legs at carpal joints and pull front legs off edge of table.

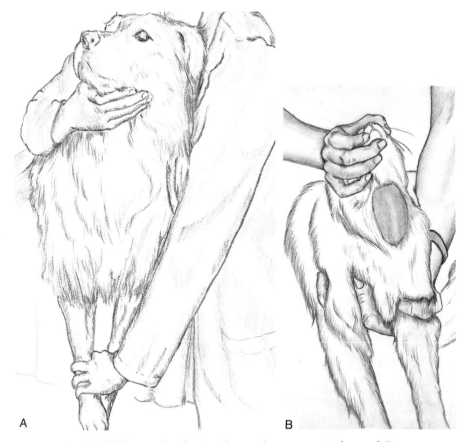

A   B

Figure 2-1 Restraint for jugular venipuncture: *A*, dog and *B*, cat.

3. With other hand, extend animal's neck by grasping its muzzle and directing its nostrils toward ceiling (Fig. 2-1).

Alternate position: Restrain animal in lateral recumbency with neck extended and front legs pulled caudally (Fig. 2-2).

> NOTE: *Whenever possible, obtain blood samples by jugular puncture.*

Position for Collection from Cephalic Vein (Fig. 2-3)

1. Place animal in sitting position or sternal recumbency.
2. Extend animal's front leg by placing fingers of one hand behind animal's elbow.
3. Compress cephalic vein with thumb and stabilize vein on dorsal surface of front leg by stretching skin slightly.

Position for Collection from Lateral Saphenous Vein (Recurrent Tarsal Vein) (Fig. 2-4)

1. Place animal in lateral recumbency.
2. Extend stifle and compress vein by firmly grasping animal's distal thigh or proximal tibial segment.

Position for Collection From Femoral Vein (Fig. 2-5)

1. Place animal in lateral recumbency.
2. With one hand, abduct uppermost hindleg to permit access to medial aspect of other hindleg.
3. With other hand, compress femoral vein on medial side of upper thigh with thumb.

> NOTE: *An additional person may be needed to restrain the head and forelegs of the animal for this procedure.*

Procedure

Technical Action	Rationale/Amplification
1. Prepare bandage for cephalic, saphenous, or femoral vein from dry cotton ball and 1-inch wide adhesive tape. Fold over tab at one end of adhesive strip.	1. Bandaging of peripheral veins following venipuncture minimizes hemorrhage and hematoma formation. Folded-over adhesive tab facilitates removal of the bandage later.
2. Swab area of vein with cotton moistened with 70% alcohol or other skin disinfectant.	2. Skin disinfectant moistens hair, making vein easier to see, and removes surface debris.

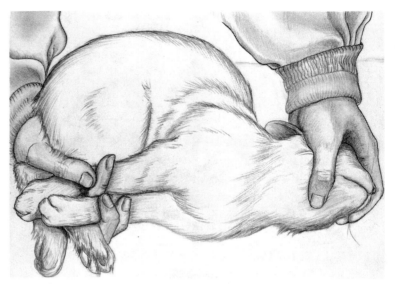

Figure 2-2 Restraint for jugular venipuncture with animal in lateral recumbency.

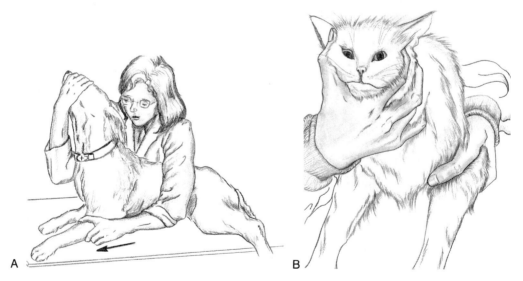

Figure 2-3 Restraint for cephalic venipuncture: (*A*) dog; (*B*) cat.

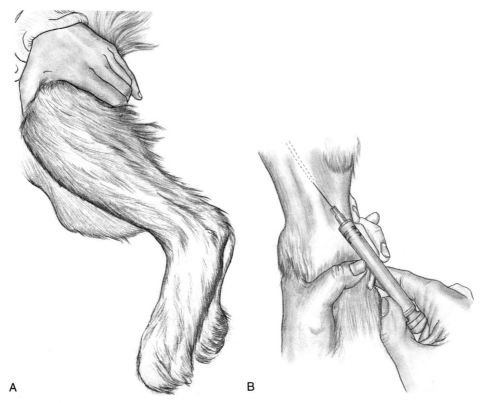

A   B

Figure 2-4 (*A* and *B*) Lateral saphenous venipuncture.

Technical Action

3. Distend vein with blood ("raise vein") by compressing vein closer to heart than venipuncture site.

4. Clip hair from area if vein cannot be seen or palpated.

Rationale/Amplification

3. The restrainer distends the vein for cephalic, saphenous, and femoral venipuncture, while the person performing venipuncture holds the leg at metacarpal/metatarsal region with one hand. The person performing jugular venipuncture distends the jugular vein with one hand by pressing firmly with thumb or fingertips on lower neck near thoracic inlet (Fig. 2-6).

4. All veins are difficult to see and palpate in obese animals. In emergency situations, a cut-down

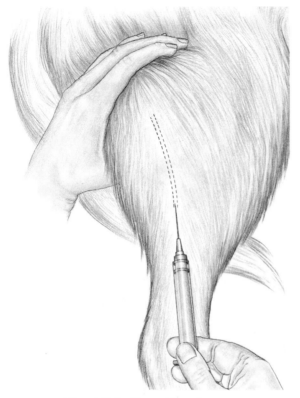

Figure 2-5   Femoral venipuncture.

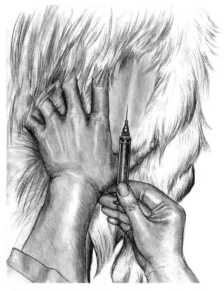

Figure 2-6   Distending jugular vein.

Technical Action	**Rationale/Amplification**
	procedure may be necessary to expose the vein. (pp. 58–61). The jugular vein is preferred for blood collection in cats and toy breed dogs because of the small size of leg veins. Hair clipping should be avoided whenever possible if the animal is exhibited regularly.
5. Select appropriate venipuncture equipment for vein and animal.	**5.** Use of appropriate equipment will help to minimize trauma to the vein. A 22-gauge needle is suitable for animals weighing up to 60 lbs; a 20-gauge needle may be used for dogs over 60 lbs in weight. The Vacutainer system

Technical Action

6. Inspect venipuncture equipment
   for flaws.

7. Hold syringe barrel or Vacutainer system so that needle
   bevel is up. Insert needle at approximately 30-degree angle
   with skin so that distal ½ inch
   of needle is threaded into vein
   (Fig. 2-7).

8. If vein rolls to either side, insert
   needle under skin lateral to vein,
   then puncture vein.

Rationale/Amplification

should not be used on small
veins because the vacuum in the
blood collection tube may cause
collapse of a small vein.

6. Discard any needles with barbed
   ends. If needle and syringe are
   to be used, attach the needle to
   the syringe and move the syringe
   plunger back and forth several
   times to determine that it moves
   freely.

7. Usually the needle can be inserted through the skin and
   directly into the vein with one
   motion. Appearance of a few
   drops of blood in the needle hub
   or at the distal end of the Vacutainer needle is evidence of successful venipuncture.

8. Rolling of the blood vessel under
   the skin is a common problem in
   certain breeds (*e.g.,* Dachshund),
   and with certain veins (*i.e.,* the
   lateral saphenous vein).

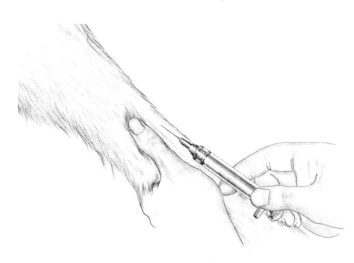

Figure 2-7 Introducing needle into
vein.

Technical Action

9. Aspirate blood by withdrawing syringe plunger. If Vacutainer system is used, force blood collection tube stopper onto distal end of needle after one or two drops of blood have appeared.

10. Release (or ask restrainer to release) distending pressure on vein.

11. Remove needle from vein and immediately apply pressure to venipuncture site with dry cotton ball.

12. Apply previously prepared bandage with some compression to cephalic, saphenous, or femoral venipuncture site (Fig. 2-9). Hold firm pressure on jugular venipuncture site for at least 60 seconds.

Rationale/Amplification

9. A needle inserted into the cephalic vein can be stabilized by holding the syringe or Vacutainer holder in place with the thumb and wrapping the fingers around the animal's leg until collection is completed (Fig. 2-8). If blood flow stops suddenly during collection, rotate the needle slightly within the vein, thereby positioning the bevel in the main stream of blood flow. For cephalic, saphenous, or femoral venipuncture, the animal's foot may be gently squeezed to stimulate venous blood return.

10. The distending pressure on the vein should be released before the needle is removed from the vein to minimize hemorrhage from the venipuncture site.

11. Pressure on the venipuncture site immediately after needle removal will decrease the possibility of hemorrhage.

12. Bandaging to prevent hemorrhage and subcutaneous hematoma formation is especially important in seriously ill animal patients because repeated venipuncture for diagnostic and therapeutic procedures may be necessary.

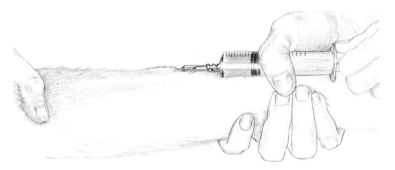

Figure 2-8 Stabilizing syringe during blood collection.

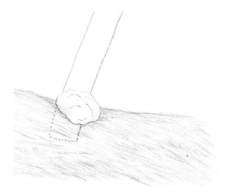

Figure 2-9 Bandaging venipuncture site after removal of needle or catheter.

Technical Action

13. Place blood promptly into appropriate collection tube(s) by allowing sample to flow into the tube. <u>When using anticoagulant coated tubes, invert blood sample gently several times to mix sample with anticoagulant.</u>

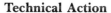

14. Remove bandage from animal's leg vein in 30 to 60 minutes.

Rationale/Amplification

13. Hemolysis of the blood sample or clotting of the blood in the syringe or anticoagulant tube can be prevented by careful handling of the sample after collection. Avoid forcefully squirting the blood through the needle into the collection tube. Vigorous shaking of a blood sample in an anticoagulant tube is more likely to result in hemolysis than is gentle inversion of the tube several times.

BLOOD COLLECTION FOR COAGULATION STUDIES

Coagulation studies are performed on venous blood.

Complications, Equipment Needed, Restraint and Positioning

As for routine venipuncture (pp. 15–17) except two syringes are required for each blood sample collected.

Procedure

Technical Action

1. Follow procedure for routine venipuncture using needle and syringe (pp. 17–22, Nos. 1 to 9).
2. Aspirate 1 ml of blood into first syringe. Leaving needle in vein, detach first syringe and discard. Attach second syringe to needle and aspirate sufficient blood for laboratory tests.
3. Follow procedure for aspirating blood, handling sample, and care of vein in routine venipuncture (pp. 22–23, Nos. 10 to 14).
4. Repeat entire procedure on normal animal.

5. If any problems occur during collection, discard sample and obtain a new sample from a different site or at a later time.

Rationale/Amplification

1. The Vacutainer system also may be used for obtaining blood for coagulation studies.
2. The two-syringe technique minimizes the amount of tissue thromboplastin in the final sample. Tissue thromboplastin released by venipuncture can alter the results of coagulation studies.

4. A control specimen should be collected by the person who collects the test sample each time coagulation studies are to be performed.
5. Blood collection problems that could affect the accuracy of coagulation studies include failure to collect a sufficient amount of blood and traumatic puncture of the skin.

ARTERIAL PUNCTURE

Arterial puncture is the placement of a needle into an artery for the purpose of obtaining a blood sample.

Purposes

To obtain a sample of arterial blood for determination of blood gaseous content and acid–base status.

Complications

1. Hemorrhage
2. Subcutaneous hematoma formation
3. Arterial thrombosis

Equipment Needed

- Cotton
- Clipper with No. 40 blade
- Skin preparation material
    Povidone–iodine surgical scrub
    Povidone–iodine solution
    Sterile gauze sponges (2″ × 2″)
- 3-ml syringe rinsed with 0.25 ml of sodium heparin (1000 USP units/ml)
- 22-gauge, 1-inch needle
- Rubber stopper
- Container of ice large enough to hold syringe

Restraint and Positioning

The femoral artery is the only superficial artery of adequate size in the dog or cat for routine arterial blood collection. The animal is placed in lateral recumbency with its uppermost hindleg abducted so that the femoral artery can be palpated on the proximal, medial aspect of the other leg.

Procedure

Technical Action	Rationale/Amplification
1. Clip hair from area.	
2. Stretch skin between thumb and forefinger of one hand and palpate femoral artery with other hand, then release while skin is prepared.	
3. Prepare skin over artery.	3. To minimize the possibility of iatrogenic infection, it is advisable to prepare the skin over the artery as if for surgery, using povidone-iodine surgical scrub and solution.
4. Inspect arterial puncture equipment (22-gauge needle and syringe) for flaws.	4. Discard any needles with barbed ends. Attach needle to syringe and move syringe plunger back and forth several times to determine that it moves freely.
5. Stretch skin between thumb and forefinger of one hand. Palpate pulsing artery proximal and distal to where skin puncture will be made.	5. Avoid contaminating exact site where arterial puncture will be performed.

Technical Action

6. Hold barrel of syringe so that needle bevel is up. Insert needle through skin at approximately 45- to 60-degree angle with the skin (Fig. 2-10).

7. Aspirate sample and remove needle from skin.

8. Hold syringe upright, tap on syringe to cause air bubbles to rise (Fig. 2-11*A*), and eject air bubbles from syringe (Fig. 2-11*B*).

9. Immediately apply firm pressure with dry cotton ball on arterial puncture site.

10. Submit sample immediately to laboratory for blood gas and pH determinations.

Rationale/Amplification

6. If possible, the needle should be inserted through the skin and directly into the artery with one motion. Successful arterial puncture has occurred if the arterial blood starts to push back the syringe plunger.

8. Evacuation of air from the syringe and insertion of needle into rubber stopper prevents inaccurate results.

9. Firm pressure on the arterial puncture site decreases the possibility of hemorrhage and subcutaneous hematoma formation. Hold pressure on arterial puncture site for 3 to 5 minutes. Hold pressure for 15 minutes or until bleeding has stopped if animal has a bleeding problem.

10. If the analysis will not be performed within 5 minutes, place the blood-filled syringe in a container with ice to preserve the condition of the blood.

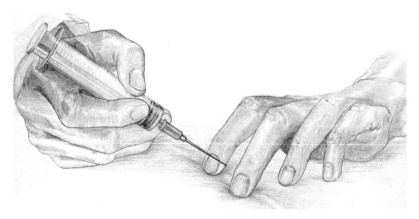

Figure 2-10 Femoral arterial puncture.

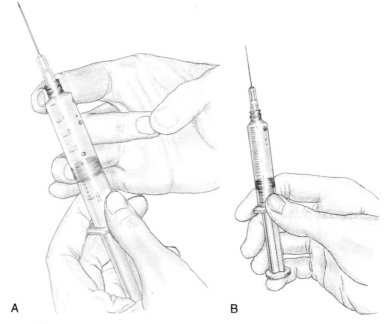

Figure 2-11 (*A* and *B*) Removing air bubbles from syringe.

TRANSFUSION COLLECTION

Transfusion collection is the obtaining of blood from a donor for use in treating a recipient.

Complications

1. Hemorrhage
2. Subcutaneous hematoma formation
3. Fibrosis of jugular vein

Equipment Needed

• Cotton
• Clipper with No. 40 blade
• Skin preparation materials
    Povidone–iodine surgical scrub
    Povidone–iodine solution
    Sterile gauze sponges (2″ × 2″)

- Drugs for sedation or anesthesia if necessary
- Bandaging material
    Sterile gauze sponges
    Antimicrobial ointment
    Gauze bandage
    Adhesive tape (2 inches wide)
- Collection apparatus for canine blood
    Vacuum bottle containing acid citrate dextrose (ACD) and donor set (16-gauge, 1½ inch needle and plastic tubing), or
    Plastic collection bag containing citrate phosphate dextrose (CPD) with accompanying needle and tubing
- Collection apparatus for feline blood
    50-ml syringe containing 7 ml of CPD, or 3 ml of sterile saline for injection and 250 USP units of sodium heparin
    18- or 21-gauge winged infusion set

Restraint and Positioning

The animal should be restrained in sternal or lateral recumbency on a table for collection from the jugular vein (Figs. 2-1 and 2-2). Sedation or administration of anesthetic may be needed because the animal must remain relatively immobile throughout the 5- to 15-minute collection procedure to minimize trauma to the jugular vein.

Procedure

Technical Action

1. Clip hair from ventral neck area.

2. Prepare ventral neck area as if for surgery, using povidone–iodine surgical scrub and solution.

3. Distend jugular vein with blood as for routine venipuncture (Fig. 2-6).

4. Insert needle (with bevel up) into jugular vein.

5. Collect sample, gently agitating collection container several times during collection.

Rationale/Amplification

1. Good visualization of the jugular vein helps prevent traumatic venipuncture.

2. Strict attention to asepsis is important to decrease the possibility of thrombophlebitis and subsequent fibrosis of the donor animal's jugular vein.

4. The needle hub may be taped loosely to the neck during collection, using 1-inch wide adhesive tape.

5. Gentle agitation of the blood collection container ensures mixing of the blood with the anticoagulant.

Technical Action

6. Release distending pressure on vein if it has been necessary to maintain distending pressure throughout collection.

7. Remove needle from vein and immediately hold pressure with dry cotton ball on venipuncture site for at least 1 minute.

8. Apply sterile bandage to neck area, with antimicrobial ointment, directly over venipuncture site.

Rationale/Amplification

6. The distending pressure on the vein should be released before the needle is removed from the vein to minimize hemorrhage from the venipuncture site.

8. Firm pressure for at least 1 minute, followed by bandaging of the neck area for at least 24 hours after transfusion collection, will help to prevent hemorrhage, subcutaneous hematoma formation, and thrombophlebitis.

Bibliography

Anderson LK: The coagulation system: Some tips on testing. Comp Contin Educ for AHT 1(5):200–205, 1980

Brunner LS, Suddarth DS: The Lippincott Manual of Nursing Practice, 3rd ed. Philadelphia, JB Lippincott, 1982

Intravartolo C: Blood transfusions in dogs and cats. Comp Contin Educ for AHT 2(6):302–308, 1981

Jones BV: Animal Nursing, Part 1. Oxford, Pergamon Press, 1966

Kirk RW, Bistner SI: Handbook of Veterinary Procedures and Emergency Treatment, 4th ed. Philadelphia, WB Saunders, 1985

Pichler ME, Turnwald GH: Blood transfusion in the dog and cat, Part I: Physiology, collection, storage, and indications for whole blood therapy. Comp Contin Educ for Prac Vet 7(1):64–71, 1985

Schall WD, Perman V: Diseases of the red blood cells. In Ettinger SJ (ed): Textbook of Veterinary Internal Medicine, Vol 2. Philadelphia, WB Saunders, 1975

Chapter 3

INJECTION TECHNIQUES

Well done is better than well said.

BENJAMIN FRANKLIN

There are five major routes by which injections can be given: intravenous (IV, within a vein), intramuscular (IM, within a muscle), subcutaneous (SC, under the skin), intraperitoneal (IP, within the peritoneal cavity), and intradermal (ID, within the skin).

Purposes

To administer fluids, pharmacologic agents, biologic preparations, and certain test substances.

The injection route that has been determined by the manufacturer to be the most effective and the safest usually is indicated on the product label. Certain materials must be administered intravenously because they will cause tissue necrosis if given outside the vascular system. Suspensions (cloudy-appearing liquids) should never be given by the intravenous or intraperitoneal routes. When no information is given regarding appropriate routes of administration, refer to guidelines in Table 3-1.

Complications

1. Irritation, necrosis, or infection at injection site
2. Allergic reaction to material injected
3. Nerve damage (mainly a complication of intramuscular injections)
4. Damage to abdominal viscera and peritonitis (a complication of intraperitoneal injections)

TABLE 3-1. Recommended Routes of Injection

Prescribed Agent	Possible Route(s)
Biologic preparations, (*e.g.*, vaccines)	Subcutaneous, intramuscular
Pharmacologic agents, (*e.g.*, antibiotics, tranquilizers)	Intravenous, intramuscular, subcutaneous, intraperitoneal
Local anesthetic agents	Intradermal, subcutaneous
Fluids	Intravenous, subcutaneous, intraperitoneal
Certain test substances	Intravenous, intramuscular, intradermal
Dialysate solutions	Intraperitoneal

Equipment Needed

- Cotton
- 70% alcohol or other skin disinfectant
- Sterile syringe of appropriate size
- Sterile needle of appropriate size
- Adhesive tape, 1 inch wide
- Clipper with No. 40 blade
- Skin preparation materials (for intraperitoneal injections)
    Povidone–iodine surgical scrub
    Povidone–iodine solution
    Sterile gauze sponges (2″ × 2″)

Restraint and Positioning

The degree of restraint required depends on the temperament of the animal and the route of injection. It is helpful to have an assistant restrain the animal, although this may not be necessary for subcutaneous injections in tractable animals. The animal should be positioned so that the intended injection site is accessible (Chap. 1).

PREPARATION FOR INJECTIONS

Procedure

Technical Action

1. Check medication with regard to "The Five Rights": right patient, right drug, right dose, right route, right time and frequency. Also check expiration date and examine medication for presence of foreign material.

Rationale/Amplification

1. It is important to take measures to prevent errors in medication administration.

Technical Action	**Rationale/Amplification**
2. Wash hands.	**2.** Washing hands between patients is important in controlling communicable diseases in a hospital.
3. Select appropriate needle size.	**3.** Use of appropriate needle size will help to minimize trauma to the tissues. For IV, IM, SQ, and IP injections, use 22-gauge needle for animals weighing up to 60 lbs and 20-gauge or 22-gauge needle for dogs over 60 lbs. For ID injections, use 25-gauge or 27-gauge needle.
4. Aseptically attach sterile needle to sterile syringe.	**4.** Syringe size will be dictated by volume of material to be injected, for example, a tuberculin syringe is routinely used for intradermal injections.
5. Use cotton moistened with 70% alcohol to swab rubber stopper of bottle containing material to be injected.	**5.** Cleaning the rubber stopper removes any dust or other contaminants.
6. Remove needle cover and aspirate into syringe a volume of air equal to that of the material to be injected. Inject this air into bottle.	**6.** Pressurizing multiple dose vials with air facilitates withdrawal of material to be injected.

NOTE: *Steps No. 5 and No. 6 are unnecessary if using ampules. An ampule is opened by fracturing the glass and then the contents are drawn up directly into the needle and attached syringe.*

7. Aspirate desired amount of medication by withdrawing syringe plunger.	
8. Remove needle (with attached syringe) from vial or ampule.	
9. Hold syringe vertically with needle pointing toward ceiling and move any large air bubbles to syringe nozzle by tapping syringe briskly. Release air bubbles through needle by advancing syringe plunger slightly (Fig. 2-11), p. 27.	**9.** Removing air bubbles from the syringe eliminates the risk of air embolism when the material is injected. Large air bubbles displace liquid material and could cause inaccurate dosing.

Technical Action

10. Replace needle cover until ready to administer injection.

Rationale/Amplification

10. Needle contamination must be avoided to minimize causing iatrogenic infection.

INTRAVENOUS INJECTION

Procedure

Technical Action

1. Prepare for injection.
2. Place animal in appropriate position for intravenous injection into jugular, cephalic, lateral saphenous, or femoral vein.
3. Follow procedure described for blood collection (Chapter 2, Nos. 1 to 4, pp. 17–20).

4. Hold syringe barrel so that needle bevel is up. Insert needle at approximately 30-degree angle with skin.

5. Advance needle into vein up to hub.

6. Release (or ask assistant to release) distending pressure on vein.

7. Aspirate small amount of blood into needle hub.

8. Inject material at moderate rate into vein. Stabilize needle inserted into cephalic vein by tapping syringe barrel to leg or by holding syringe barrel with thumb while wrapping fingers around animal's leg (Fig. 2-8, p. 22).

Rationale/Amplification

1. See pp. 31–33.
2. See Chapter 2, pp. 15–17.

3. Prepare bandage, disinfect venipuncture site, distend vein with blood, and clip hair (if necessary).
4. If vessel rolls, insert needle under skin lateral to the vein, then puncture the vein. Appearance of a few drops of blood in the needle hub is evidence of successful venipuncture.
5. When syringe plunger is withdrawn, blood should flow quickly into syringe.
6. The distending pressure must be released to allow the injected material to flow easily into the circulation.
7. A rapid flow of blood into the syringe is assurance of proper needle placement.
8. When a volume greater than 5 ml or when any irritating substance is injected intravenously, it is advisable to check needle placement within the vein by aspirating blood into the syringe several times during the injection.

Technical Action

9. Remove needle from vein and immediately apply pressure with dry cotton ball to venipuncture site.

10. Apply previously prepared bandage with some compression to cephalic, saphenous, or femoral venipuncture site. Hold firm pressure on jugular venipuncture site for at least 60 seconds.

11. Note on animal's medical record that medication was given.

12. Remove bandage from animal's leg in 30 to 60 minutes.

Rationale/Amplification

9. Pressure on the venipuncture site immediately following needle removal will decrease the possibility of hemorrhage and perivascular leakage of the injected material.

10. Bandaging to prevent hemorrhage and subcutaneous hematoma formation is especially important in seriously ill animal patients because repeated venipuncture for diagnostic and therapeutic procedures may be necessary.

11. Note date, time, medication, serial/lot number, dosage, route, initials of person administering medication, and comments.

INTRAMUSCULAR INJECTION

Procedure

only a 1 in. needle

Technical Action

1. Prepare for injection.
2. Place animal in lateral recumbency or in sitting or standing position.

Rationale/Amplification

1. See pp. 31–33.
2. Intramuscular injections are given in the quadriceps muscle group on anterior thigh, lumbodorsal muscles on either side of lumbar vertebrae, or triceps muscles, posterior to humerus in front leg (Fig. 3-1). All three of the recommended muscle groups can be used when the animal is sitting, standing, or in lateral or sternal recumbency. The hamstring muscle group (semitendinosus, semimembranosus) should be avoided if at all possible because of the risk of sciatic nerve injury.

– go in at an angle; you will not damage nerves.

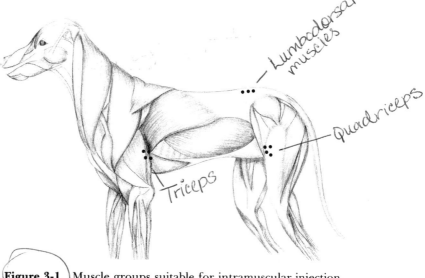

Lumbodorsal muscles

Quadriceps

Triceps

Figure 3-1 Muscle groups suitable for intramuscular injection.

Technical Action

3. Restrain animal as needed.

4. Swab skin over intended injection site with cotton moistened with 70% alcohol or other skin disinfectant.

5. Insert needle through skin into muscle at approximately 45-degree to 90-degree angle (Fig. 3-2).

6. Before injecting, pull back on syringe plunger. If blood enters syringe, select a different injection site in another muscle or a different part of same muscle.

7. If no blood is aspirated into syringe, inject material at moderate rate into muscle.

Rationale/Amplification

3. Intramuscular injections can be painful.

4. A disinfectant removes surface debris from the skin and hair.

5. Quick insertion of the needle through muscle tissue is less painful than slow advancement of the needle.

6. The presence of blood in the syringe indicates that a blood vessel has been entered. Some agents, approved for intramuscular use only, may cause severe allergic reactions and even death if given intravascularly.

7. The maximum volume that should be injected intramuscularly at any one site is 2 ml in the cat and 3 ml to 5 ml in the dog. Muscle tissue is dense and cannot accommodate large volumes of injectable material.

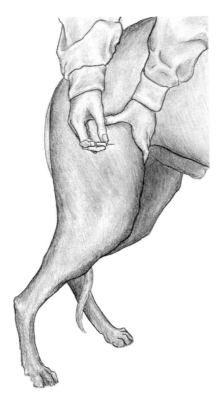

Figure 3-2   Placement of needle for intramuscular injection into quadriceps.

Technical Action

8. Remove needle from muscle and gently massage muscle.

9. Note in animal's medical record that medication was given.

Rationale/Amplification

8. Massaging the muscle after injection aids in dispersal of the injected material and decreases pain.

9. Note date, time, medication, serial/lot number, dosage, route, initials, and comments. It is important to note the injection site so that the available sites can be rotated during subsequent intramuscular injections.

SUBCUTANEOUS INJECTION

Procedure

Technical Action

1. Prepare for injection.
2. Place animal in sternal recumbency, or in standing or sitting position.
3. Pick up fold of skin over animal's neck or back by pinching skin between thumb and fingers.
4. Swab skin over intended injection site with cotton moistened with 70% alcohol or other skin disinfectant.
5. Insert needle to its hub through skin fold into subcutaneous tissue space (Fig. 3-3).

6. Before injecting, pull back on syringe plunger and observe if any blood enters syringe. If blood enters syringe, select a different injection site.

Rationale/Amplification

1. See pp. 31–33.
2. Most cats and dogs tolerate subcutaneous injections quite well so that minimal restraint is required.
3. Cats and dogs have freely movable skin along the dorsal portion of the neck and back.
4. A disinfectant removes surface debris from the skin and hair.

5. The needle should slide easily under the skin. If resistance is met, the needle may be positioned intradermally or intramuscularly and should be redirected.
6. The presence of blood in the syringe indicates that a blood vessel has been entered. Some agents, approved for subcutaneous use only, may cause severe allergic reactions and even death if given intravascularly.

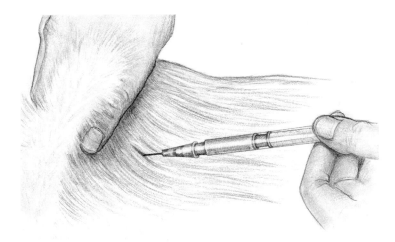

Figure 3-3 Placement of needle for subcutaneous injection.

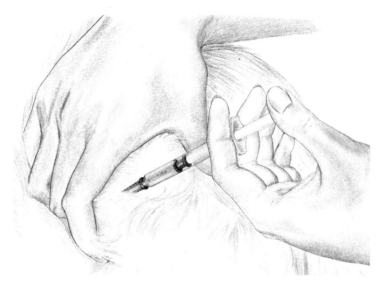

Figure 3-4   Subcutaneous injection.

Technical Action

7. If no blood can be aspirated into syringe, inject material at moderate rate under skin (Fig. 3-4).

8. Remove needle from skin and massage injection area.

9. Note in animal's medical record that medication was given.

Rationale/Amplification

7. The dorsal subcutaneous tissue of dogs and cats can accommodate relatively large volumes of fluid, from 30 ml to 50 ml at one site.

8. Massaging the injection site aids in dispersal of the injected material.

9. Note date, time, medication, serial/lot number, dosage, route, initials, and comments.

INTRAPERITONEAL INJECTION

Procedure

Technical Action

1. Prepare for injection.
2. Select an appropriate gauge and length needle.

Rationale/Amplification

1. See pp. 31–33.
2. The needle used for intraperitoneal injections should be 1½ inches to 3 inches in length. An over-the-needle intravenous catheter may be used instead of a needle for this procedure.

Technical Action	**Rationale/Amplification**
3. Palpate the abdomen to determine whether the urinary bladder is empty.	**3.** If the animal's bladder is empty, the possibility of inadvertently puncturing this organ is markedly reduced. If the bladder is distended, allow the animal to urinate or empty bladder by catheterization.
4. Place animal in dorsal or lateral recumbency.	**4.** Depending on the animal's size and temperament, one or two assistants will be needed to restrain the animal.
5. Clip hair over central abdomen and prepare skin as for surgery, using povidone–iodine surgical scrub and solution (Chap. 16, pp. 141–142).	**5.** Adequate preparation of the skin will help to decrease the possibility of peritonitis resulting from this procedure.
6. Elevate animal's hindquarters approximately 4 to 6 inches higher than front quarters.	**6.** Elevation of the hindquarters allows most of the viscera to move anterior to the intended injection site.
7. Insert needle at a point midway between umbilicus and pubis just lateral to linea alba (Fig. 3-5).	**7.** Direct needle toward pubis into abdomen.

full —

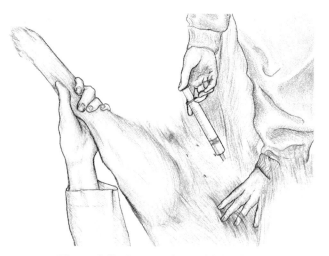

Figure 3-5   Intraperitoneal injection.

Technical Action

8. Before injecting, pull back on syringe plunger and observe for blood, urine, or intestinal contents entering syringe.

9. If blood, urine, or intestinal contents are not aspirated into syringe, inject material at moderate rate into peritoneal cavity.
10. Remove needle from abdomen.
11. Note in animal's medical record that medication was given.

Rationale/Amplification

8. The presence of blood, urine, or intestinal contents in the syringe indicates that the needle is positioned incorrectly within the peritoneal cavity or that there is abdominal disease or injury.
9. The peritoneal cavity of dogs and cats can accommodate relatively large volumes of fluid (*e.g.*, up to 6 liters in a large dog).

11. Note date, time, medication, serial/lot number, dosage route, initials, and comments.

INTRADERMAL INJECTION

Procedure

Technical Action

1. Prepare for injection.
2. Clip hair for injections.

3. Avoid use of soaps or disinfectants on skin where intradermal skin test injections will be made.
4. For intradermal skin testing, place animal in lateral recumbency.
5. Mark skin beneath each intended injection site with felt-tip pen.

6. Hold syringe barrel with needle bevel up at approximately 10-degree angle with skin.

Rationale/Amplification

1. See pp. 31–33.
2. For a single injection, clip about a 4-inch square area on lateral abdomen or thorax. For intradermal skin testing, clip a large area on the thorax or abdomen. Clipping should be done in an area that is free of skin lesions. Gentle use of the clippers is essential to avoid trauma to the skin.
3. Such agents may cause local allergic reactions that will mask test results.

5. Marking ensures even spacing of injections and facilitates recording of test results.

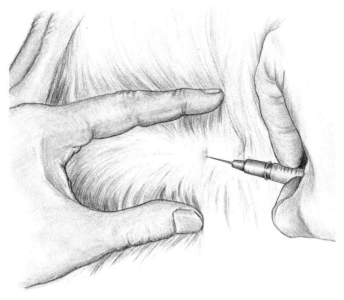

Figure 3-6   Inserting needle intradermally.

Technical Action

7. Stretch skin between thumb and forefinger of one hand and insert needle within epidermis until bevel is completely enclosed within skin layers (Fig. 3-6).

8. Check for correct placement of needle intradermally by lifting up on tip of needle.

9. Inject 0.05 to 0.1 ml intradermally (Fig. 3-7); then remove needle from skin.

10. For intradermal infiltration of local anesthetic agent, place animal in position that affords access to area to be injected.

11. Clip hair from area to be infiltrated with local anesthetic and prepare skin, using povidone-iodine surgical scrub and solution (Chap. 16, pp. 141–142).

Rationale/Amplification

7. It is not necessary to insert the needle to its hub when giving an intradermal injection.

8. The metal of the needle should be just visible through the epidermis if the needle is positioned properly.

9. A small intradermal bleb of fluid should be present at the injection site.

10. Local anesthesia may be used for excision of small benign skin lesions and suturing of small wounds.

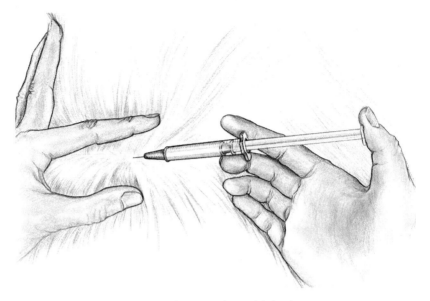

Figure 3-7 Intradermal injection.

Technical Action	**Rationale/Amplification**
12. Inject local anesthetic intradermally, repeating Nos. 6 to 8, pp. 40–41.	**12.** The volume of local anesthetic used will depend on the size and location of the lesion.

Bibliography

Brunner LS, Suddarth DS: The Lippincott Manual of Nursing Practice, 3rd ed. Philadelphia, JB Lippincott, 1982

Kirk RW, Bistner SI: Handbook of Veterinary Procedures and Emergency Treatment, 4th ed. Philadelphia, WB Saunders, 1985

Pratt PW (ed): Medical Nursing for Animal Health Technicians. Santa Barbara, American Veterinary Publications, 1985

Chapter 4

Rd.
for Wed.

PLACEMENT AND CARE OF INTRAVENOUS CATHETERS

The recollection of quality remains long after the price has been forgotten.

BENJAMIN FRANKLIN

Intravenous catheterization is the placement of a hollow device, a catheter, into a vein.

Purposes

1. To administer fluids, medication, anesthetic agents, blood, and certain test substances
2. To monitor central venous pressure

Complications

1. Occlusion, malpositioning, and breakage of the catheter
2. Thrombophlebitis
3. Infiltration of subcutaneous tissues
4. Infection
5. Hemorrhage and subcutaneous hematoma formation
6. Pyrogenic reaction
7. Circulatory overload
8. Air embolism
9. Allergic reaction

Equipment Needed

- Cotton
- Clipper with No. 40 blade
- Skin preparation materials
    Povidone–iodine surgical scrub
    Povidone–iodine solution
    Sterile gauze sponges ($2'' \times 2''$)
- Bandaging material
    Sterile gauze sponges
    Antimicrobial ointment
    Gauze bandage
    Adhesive tape ($1/2''$, $1''$, and $2''$)
    Splint (if necessary)
- Syringe containing 1 ml of heparinized saline (500 IU sodium heparin in 250 ml of normal saline)
- Injection cap
- Fluid administration set (if necessary)
- Extension tubing (if necessary)
- Intravenous catheter
    Winged infusion set ("butterfly")
    Over-the-needle catheter ("needle inside")
    Through-the-needle catheter ("needle outside")

Restraint and Positioning

There are four veins in both dogs and cats that are accessible for intravenous catheterization: jugular, cephalic, lateral saphenous (recurrent tarsal), and femoral. The jugular is the vein of choice for administration of hypertonic solutions, long-term fluid administration, and central venous pressure measurement.

Adequate restraint is important throughout the procedure to ensure aseptic placement of the catheter and proper bandaging of the catheterization site. The position used depends on the vein selected for catheterization. (See Chap. 2, pp. 16–17).

PREPARATION FOR INTRAVENOUS CATHETERIZATION

Procedure

Technical Action

1. Wash hands.

2. Clip hair over a wide area around the insertion site.

Rationale/Amplification

1. Every precaution must be taken to reduce the chance of causing iatrogenic infection.

2. Good visualization of the vein aids in atraumatic venipuncture. Clip-

Technical Action

3. Prepare clipped area as if for surgery, using povidone–iodine surgical scrub and solution (Chap. 16, pp. 141–142).

4. Select intravenous catheter of appropriate diameter and length (Table 4-1).

5. Inspect catheter for flaws.

Rationale/Amplification

ping of hair is a necessary part of adequate skin preparation.

4. Factors influencing catheter selection include size and location of vein and the reason for catheterization. To minimize thrombophlebitis, use the smallest diameter catheter that will allow the infusion rate required to meet a particular animal's needs.

5. Discard any catheter with a barbed needle or with immobile parts.

TABLE 4-1. Recommended Intravenous Catheter Sizes for Routine Use in Dogs and Cats

Animal	Vein	Catheter Type	Size
Cat	Cephalic	Over-the-needle	20 gauge, 1½ in
	Femoral	Over-the-needle	20 gauge, 1½ in
	Jugular	Through-the-needle	19-gauge catheter, 8 in
Dog	Cephalic	Through-the-needle	19-gauge catheter, 8 or 12 in
		Over-the-needle	18- or 20-gauge, 1½ in
	Lateral saphenous	Through-the-needle	19-gauge catheter, 8 or 12 in
		Over-the-needle	18- or 20-gauge, 1½ in
	Jugular (≤ 65 lb)	Through-the-needle	19-gauge catheter, 8 or 12 in
	Jugular (> 65 lb)	Through-the-needle	16-gauge catheter, 12 in

INSERTION OF WINGED INFUSION SET ("BUTTERFLY")

Procedure

Technical Action

1. Prepare for catheterization.

Rationale/Amplification

1. See pp. 44–45. The relatively short needle on the winged infusion set limits its use, for the most part, to cephalic, saphenous, and femoral veins.

Technical Action

2. Distend (or ask assistant to distend) vein with blood.
3. Hold winged infusion set so that bevel of needle is up, while squeezing wings of set together between thumb and index finger (Fig. 4-1).
4. Insert needle (with bevel up) at approximately 30-degree angle with skin.
5. Advance needle into vein.

6. Release (or ask assistant to release) distending pressure on vein.
7. Attach injection cap, syringe, or fluid infusion set, and begin administration of prescribed fluid or agent.

Rationale/Amplification

2. See Chap. 2, p. 19, No. 3.

3. In general, insertion of a needle into a vein with its bevel up helps to minimize trauma to the wall of the vein.

4. A flash of blood should appear in the plastic tubing near the proximal end of the needle.
5. Inadvertent puncturing of the opposite wall of the vein usually can be avoided by lifting the wings slightly while threading the needle into the vein.

7. Starting the infusion helps to anchor the needle in the vein and prevent backflow of blood. In general, winged infusion sets

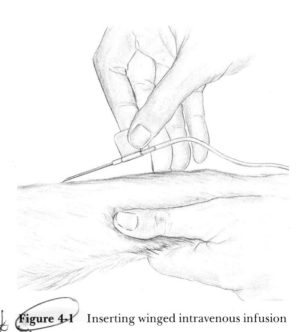

Figure 4-1 Inserting winged intravenous infusion set.

Technical Action

Rationale/Amplification

are suitable in animals only for short-term administration of pharmacologic agents or for fluid administration during anesthesia. An injection cap is not required under these circumstances.

8. Hold infusion set in place by applying adhesive tape parallel to needle on each wing, then across entire apparatus and encircling leg (Fig. 4-2).

8. The tape serves to hold the needle in place.

9. Make loop in tubing and tape this loop to animal (Fig. 4-2).

9. If the animal moves, the butterfly needle can easily become dislodged or puncture the opposite wall of the vein. A loop in the tubing prevents traction on the needle when the leg and infusion set are moved.

10. Continued position of butterfly needle within vein can be checked by aspiration of blood into a syringe or by lowering fluid bottle below animal's body level.

10. Frequent checking of correct needle placement is advisable when irritating substances are being administered through a winged infusion set.

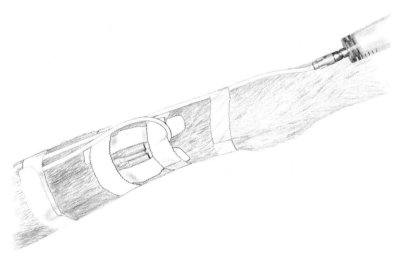

Figure 4-2 Securing winged intravenous infusion set and intravenous tubing.

Technical Action

11. Remove needle from vein and immediately apply pressure to venipuncture site with dry cotton ball.

12. Apply previously prepared bandage with gentle compression to cephalic, saphenous, or femoral venipuncture site (Fig. 2-9, p. 23). Maintain firm pressure on jugular venipuncture site for at least 60 seconds.

13. Remove bandage from animal's leg vein in 30 to 60 minutes.

Rationale/Amplification

11. Pressure on the venipuncture site and bandaging of the site following needle removal will decrease the possibility of hemorrhage and subcutaneous hematoma formation.

12. Bandaging to prevent hemorrhage and subcutaneous hematoma formation is especially important in seriously ill animal patients because repeated venipuncture for diagnostic and therapeutic procedures may be necessary.

INSERTION OF OVER-THE-NEEDLE CATHETER ("NEEDLE INSIDE")

Procedure

Technical Action

1. Prepare for catheterization.

2. Place sufficient length of 1/2-inch adhesive tape around catheter hub to encircle animal's leg.

3. Distend (or ask assistant to distend) vein with blood.

4. Insert needle and catheter into vein with needle bevel up (Fig. 4-3).

5. Advance needle into vein until at least 1/2 inch of needle is within vein.

Rationale/Amplification

1. See pp. 44–45. Over-the-needle catheters are not recommended for use in the jugular vein. The short length of these catheters impedes securing them in the neck. Also it is difficult to puncture the thicker skin in the neck area with an over-the-needle catheter.

2. This tape will serve to anchor the catheter firmly to the leg once it has been placed in the vein.

3. See Chap. 2, p. 19, No. 3.

4. Rapid flow of blood into the hub of the needle indicates successful venipuncture.

5. The catheter is slightly shorter than the needle in an over-the-needle catheter. Entry of the

Technical Action

Rationale/Amplification

catheter into the lumen of the vein is ensured by placing the distal 1/2 inch of the needle within the lumen of the vein.

6. Hold needle in place and slowly advance only the catheter farther into vein until catheter hub is at point of skin puncture (Fig. 4-4). If the catheter will not thread easily, remove entire apparatus, place a temporary bandage over the venipuncture site, and attempt catheterization in another vein or at a more proximal part of the same vein.

6. Once the advancing of the catheter has begun, the metal needle must not be reinserted through the catheter because the needle could cut the catheter.

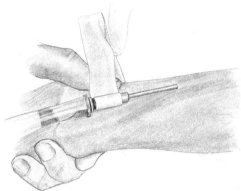

Figure 4-3 Inserting over-the-needle intravenous catheter.

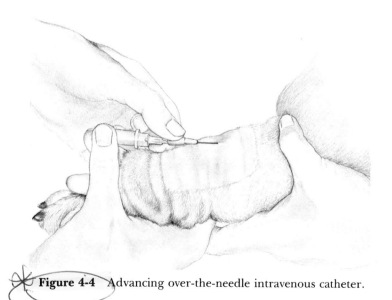

Figure 4-4 Advancing over-the-needle intravenous catheter.

Technical Action

7. Hold catheter hub and withdraw needle from catheter.

8. Place injection cap on catheter (Fig. 4-5).

9. Wrap adhesive tape strip attached to catheter hub around animal's leg.

10. Flush catheter with heparinized saline.

11. Cleanse venipuncture site of any blood with cotton.

12. Place small amount of antimicrobial ointment at insertion point of catheter into skin and cover with sterile gauze sponge (Fig. 4-6).

Rationale/Amplification

7. The catheter can be removed inadvertently if it is not held in place while the needle is withdrawn.

8. An injection cap provides a sterile seal to the intravenous catheter. A needle attached to a syringe or intravenous fluid infusion tubing can be inserted through the injection cap.

9. This tape anchors the catheter to the leg. Firm anchoring of the catheter prevents trauma to the vein caused by excessive movement of the catheter.

10. Heparinized saline will keep the catheter patent while the bandage is placed on the leg.

11. Blood is a good culture medium for bacterial growth. Removal of any blood extravasated during the procedure will help to decrease the possibility of infection.

12. Local application of antimicrobial ointment is vital for preventing catheter-associated infections.

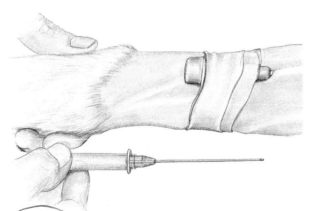

Figure 4-5 Injection cap on intravenous catheter.

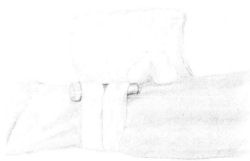

Figure 4-6 Antimicrobial ointment at insertion point of intravenous catheter into skin.

Technical Action

13. Bandage leg using gauze bandaging material and adhesive tape, leaving only the injection cap exposed (Fig. 4-7).

14. Flush catheter with heparinized saline every 8 to 12 hours when not in continuous use.

15. Remove bandage and inspect leg every 48 hours, or immediately if animal gives evidence of pain in catheterized leg, or if intravenous infusion cannot be administered easily.

Rationale/Amplification

13. Careful bandaging of the leg over a wide area helps to prevent contamination of the catheter insertion site and resulting infection. A splint may be incorporated into the bandage if the animal repeatedly moves its leg into a position that interferes with the flow rate of the intravenous infusion.

14. The heparinized saline will keep the catheter patent.

15. The bandage should be changed immediately if it becomes wet or soiled. Every 48 hours, the bandage should be changed and the leg inspected for swelling, pain, redness, or increased skin temperature. Such signs may indicate one or more of the following complications: infiltration of subcutaneous tissues due to catheter moving out of the vein, thrombophlebitis, or infection. If any of these signs are present, the catheter should be removed and the catheter tip should be submitted for bacteriologic culture.

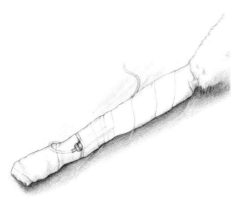

Figure 4-7 Bandage protecting intravenous catheterization site.

Technical Action

16. If continuous intravenous fluid administration is maintained, change fluid administration set and needle every 24 hours and clean injection cap with 70% alcohol.

17. When catheter is removed, immediately apply pressure to catheterization site with dry cotton ball. Then apply previously prepared bandage.

Rationale/Amplification

16. Changing the fluid administration apparatus helps to prevent the infusion of microorganisms originating within the apparatus itself.

17. Pressure on the venipuncture site and bandaging of the site following catheter removal will decrease the possibility of hemorrhage and subcutaneous hematoma formation.

INSERTION OF THROUGH-THE-NEEDLE CATHETER ("NEEDLE OUTSIDE")

Procedure

Technical Action

1. Prepare for catheterization.

2. Distend (or ask assistant to distend) vein with blood.

3. Insert needle (with catheter withdrawn inside needle) into vein with needle bevel up (Fig. 4-8).

Rationale/Amplification

1. See pp. 44–45. Examine the apparatus carefully to determine that the catheter moves easily within the needle.

2. See Chap. 2, p. 19, No. 3.

3. Because of the length of this type of catheter (8 or 12 inches), it should be inserted close to the carpus if the cephalic vein is

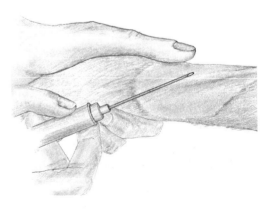

Figure 4-8 Inserting through-the-needle intravenous catheter into cephalic vein.

Technical Action

Rationale/Amplification

used. A through-the-needle catheter is inserted downward into the jugular vein toward the thoracic inlet (Fig. 4-9). It may be easier, especially in the neck area, to insert the needle through the skin before venipuncture is attempted.

4. Advance needle into vein until at least 1/2 inch of needle is within vein.

4. Venipuncture is confirmed when a flash of blood is seen in the catheter. Entry of the catheter into the lumen of the vein is ensured by placing the distal 1/2 inch of the needle within the vein before the catheter is threaded into the vein.

5. Hold needle firmly with one hand and thread catheter into vein by pushing catheter hub within plastic sleeve (Fig. 4-10A) until catheter hub has been advanced into needle hub (Fig. 4-10B).

5. Occasionally the animal's leg or neck must be flexed or extended to allow the catheter to advance as far as possible into the vein.

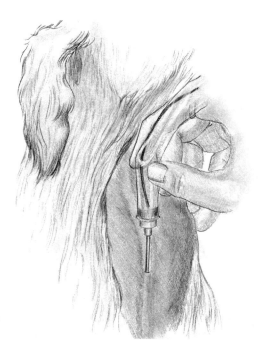

Figure 4-9 Inserting through-the-needle intravenous catheter into jugular vein.

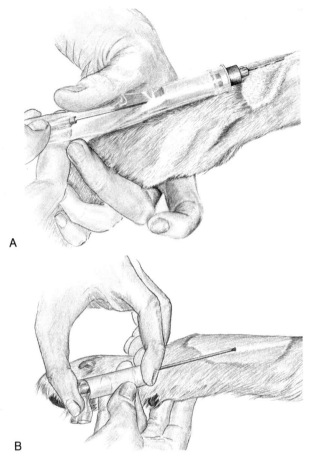

A

B

Figure 4-10 (*A*) Advancing through-the-needle intravenous catheter inside plastic sleeve, and (*B*) catheter hub fully advanced into needle hub.

Technical Action	**Rationale/Amplification**
6. Disconnect plastic sleeve from needle (Fig. 4-11).	**6.** It is sometimes necessary to hold the needle hub with a forceps to prevent excessive needle motion and possible laceration of the vein.
7. Withdraw needle from skin and remove wire stylet.	**7.** The function of the wire stylet is to add rigidity to the catheter while it is being advanced into the vein.
8. Place injection cap on catheter.	**8.** An injection cap provides a sterile seal to the catheter. A needle attached to a syringe or intraven-

Technical Action

Rationale/Amplification

ous fluid infusion tubing can be inserted through the injection cap.

9. Flush catheter with heparinized saline.

9. The heparinized saline will keep the catheter patent while the catheterization site is bandaged.

10. Place needle guard over point at which catheter emerges from tip of needle (Fig. 4-12) and snap it shut.

10. The needle guard protects the catheter from being severed by the needle.

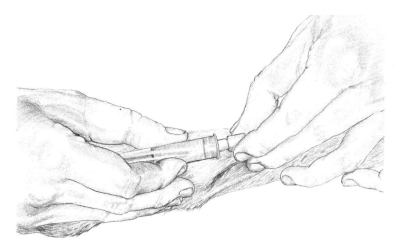

Figure 4-11   Disconnecting plastic sleeve from needle hub.

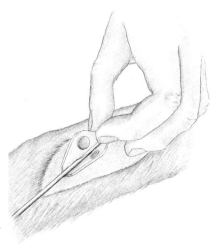

Figure 4-12   Placing needle guard on through-the-needle intravenous catheter.

Technical Action

11. Double back external portion of catheter to facilitate bandaging (Fig. 4-13).
12. Follow complete bandage procedures previously described for bandaging, care, and removal of catheter (Fig. 4-14). (See pp. 50–52, Nos. 11 to 17.)
13. If hypertonic fluids are to be administered, radiograph thorax to check catheter position within jugular vein.

Rationale/Amplification

11. Be careful not to kink the catheter.

13. It is important to make sure that the catheter is not malpositioned (*e.g.,* folded back on itself or positioned in a small vein such as the internal thoracic vein). Hypertonic solutions should be given only in large veins, where the volume of blood will decrease the possibility of thrombophlebitis.

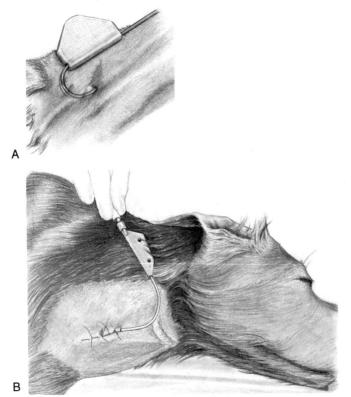

A

B

Figure 4-13 Positioning external portion of through-the-needle intravenous catheter prior to bandaging: (*A*) leg and (*B*) neck.

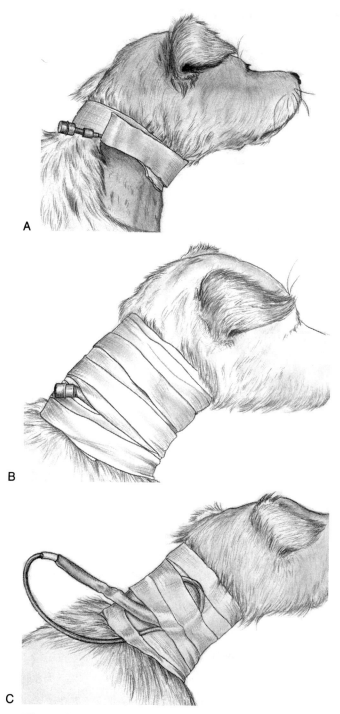

Figure 4-14 (A), (B), (C), Bandaging intravenous through-the-needle catheter in jugular vein.

INSERTION OF CUT-DOWN CATHETER

Additional Equipment Needed

- Sterile drapes
- Surgeon's gloves
- Cap and mask
- Scalpel blade
- Curved hemostat
- Suture material
    3-0 or 4-0 chromic gut for vein
    3-0 or 4-0 monofilament nonabsorbable suture material for skin
- Local anesthetic (2% lidocaine)

Procedure

Technical Action	Rationale/Amplification
1. Prepare for catheterization of the jugular vein.	1. A through-the-needle catheter is suitable for use in the cut-down procedure. In hypotensive, debilitated, or very young animals, the veins may not be visible or palpable, rendering a cut-down procedure necessary for intravenous catheterization.
2. Don cap, mask, and sterile gloves. Place sterile drapes around catheterization site.	2. Strict attention to asepsis is essential to decrease the possibility of infection.
3. Infiltrate region of incision with local anesthetic (2% lidocaine).	3. General anesthesia should be avoided because of the critical condition of the patient.
4. Make a longitudinal skin incision over jugular vein.	
5. Using blunt dissection, isolate vein and use curved hemostat to preplace two 5-inch lengths of suture material (chromic gut) under vein on each side of proposed insertion site (Fig. 4-15).	5. These ligatures will be needed above and below the venipuncture site to prevent hemorrhage. The normal compressing effect of the surrounding tissues will be disrupted by the surgical dissection.
6. Tie distal ligature (ligature closer to animal's head) but do not cut ends of ligature yet.	
7. Insert through-the-needle catheter into vein routinely but *do not remove wire stylet.*	7. See pp. 52–54 (Nos. 3 to 6).

Technical Action

8. Ligate vein around catheter proximal to insertion site (Fig. 4-16).

9. Tie loose ends of distal ligature around catheter to hold it to outside wall of vein distal to insertion site (Fig. 4-17).

Rationale/Amplification

8. The wire stylet prevents the ligature from crushing the catheter.

9. This serves to stabilize the catheter further and prevent kinking at the insertion site.

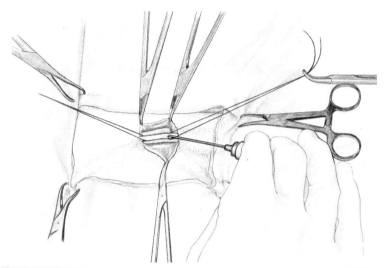

Figure 4-15 Preplacing suture material during cut-down intravenous catheterization.

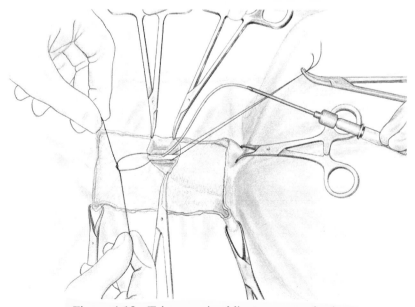

Figure 4-16 Tying proximal ligature around vein.

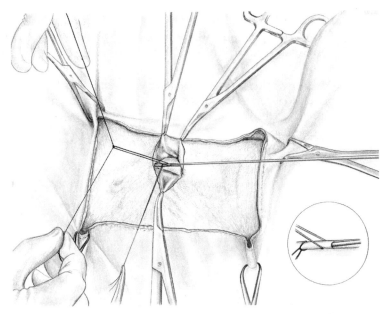

Figure 4-17   Tying distal ligature around vein and catheter.

Technical Action

10. Remove wire stylet.

11. Place injection cap on catheter.

12. Flush catheter with heparinized saline.

13. Place needle guard over point at which catheter emerges from tip of needle, and snap it shut.

14. Suture skin incision.

15. Double back external portion of catheter to facilitate bandaging (Fig. 4-13, p. 56).

16. Follow complete bandage procedure previously described for bandaging, care, and removal of catheter. (Fig. 4-14, p. 57 and pp. 50–52, Nos. 11 to 17).

Rationale/Amplification

11. An injection cap provides a sterile seal to the catheter.

12. The heparinized saline will keep the catheter patent while the skin incision is sutured and the catheterization site is bandaged.

13. The needle guard protects the catheter from being severed by the needle.

14. The skin sutures can be removed when the incision has healed (7–10 days).

15. Be careful not to kink the catheter.

Technical Action	Rationale/Amplification
17. If hypertonic fluids are to be administered, take thoracic radiograph to check catheter position within jugular vein.	**17.** It is important to make sure that the catheter is not malpositioned (*e.g.*, folded back on itself or positioned in a small vein such as the internal thoracic vein). Hypertonic solutions should be given only in large veins, where the volume of blood will decrease the possibility of thrombophlebitis.

Certain complications of intravenous therapy, such as pyrogenic reaction, circulatory overload, and air embolism, are beyond the scope of this book but are discussed in depth in *The Lippincott Manual of Nursing Practice,* third edition.

Bibliography

Brunner, LS, Suddarth DS: The Lippincott Manual of Nursing Practice, 3rd ed. Philadelphia, JB Lippincott, 1982

Burrows CF: Techniques and complications of intravenous and intraarterial catheterization in dogs and cats. JAVMA 163(12):1357–1363, 1973

Haskins SC: Fluid and electrolyte therapy. Comp Contin Educ for Pract Vet 6(3):244–257, 1984

Kirk RW, Bistner SI: Handbook of Veterinary Procedures and Emergency Treatment, 4th ed. Philadelphia, WB Saunders, 1985

Managing IV Therapy, A Nursing Photobook, In Nursing '81 Photobook. Springhouse, PA, Intermed Communications, 1980

Chapter 5

ORAL ADMINISTRATION OF MEDICATIONS

The patient man shows much good sense, but the quick-tempered man displays folly at its height.

PROVERBS 14:29

Oral administration of medications is the placement of solid or liquid material in the oral cavity so that specific quantities of the material are swallowed.

Purposes

1. To administer medications, water, and nutritional supplements
2. To administer certain radiographic contrast materials

Contraindications

1. Dysphagia, regurgitation, and vomiting
2. Acute pancreatitis
3. Esophageal and gastrointestinal obstruction
4. Esophageal surgery within the past 2 to 7 days, depending on extent of injury
5. Gastric or intestinal surgery within the past 12 to 24 hours
6. Head and neck trauma

Complications

1. Aspiration of medications into respiratory tract
2. Inaccurate dosing

Equipment Needed

- For capsules or tablets
  Lubricant
  Forceps (when indicated)
- For liquids
  Syringe, small bottle, or spoon

Restraint and Positioning

The procedure may be accomplished with the animal standing, sitting, or in sternal recumbency. Minimal restraint should be used. When handling vicious animals, oral medication can be offered in small amounts of palatable food. It is imperative that the animal be fully conscious whenever medications are administered orally.

ADMINISTRATION OF CAPSULE OR TABLET

Procedure

Technical Action	Rationale/Amplification
1. Check medication to be administered with regard to "The Five Rights": right patient, right drug, right dose, right route, right time and frequency.	1. It is important to take measures to prevent errors of medication administration.
2. Wash hands.	2. Washing hands between patients is important in controlling communicable diseases in a hospital. It is advisable to wear nonsterile examination gloves when administering oral medication to an animal with a communicable disease.
3. Lubricate capsule or tablet.	3. Lubrication of the capsule or tablet, for example, with butter or water-soluble lubricant, makes it easier to swallow.
4. Hold capsule or tablet between forceps jaws (Fig. 5-1) or thumb and index finger of one hand (Fig. 5-2).	4. A forceps is useful for administering capsules or tablets to a cat or a dog that resists attempts to hold the mouth open during the procedure.

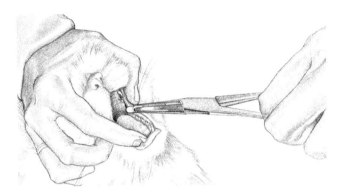

Figure 5-1 Use of forceps to hold capsule or tablet.

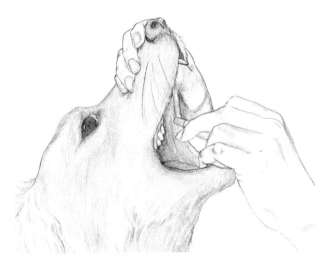

Figure 5-2 Placing capsule on base of animal's tongue.

Technical Action	**Rationale/Amplification**
5. Place palm of other hand on dorsal surface of animal's snout.	
6. Insert thumb behind one upper canine tooth into mouth and stroke the animal's hard palate.	6. Rolling the animal's lips inward over its teeth may minimize the possibility of the person being bitten. Tactile stimulation of the hard palate often leads to spontaneous opening of the mouth.
7. Tilt animal's nostrils toward ceiling.	7. This head position causes relaxation of the lower jaw muscles in

Technical Action	Rationale/Amplification
	many animals, thereby eliminating the need for forceful attempts to pry open the animal's mouth.
8. Press downward on animal's lower incisors with third, fourth, and fifth fingers of hand holding medications.	8. At this point, the animal's mouth should be open wide.
9. Place capsule or tablet on base of animal's tongue (Figs. 5-1 and 5-2).	9. An animal can easily eject from its mouth a capsule or tablet placed on the rostral portion of the tongue.
10. Withdraw hand from animal's mouth.	
11. Close animal's mouth quickly and hold it closed, while at the same time rubbing the ventral neck area.	11. Licking of the nasal planum indicates that the animal has swallowed.
12. Note in animal's medical record that medication was given.	12. The following information should be noted in the medical record: date, time, medication, dosage, route, initials of individual administering medication, and comments.

ADMINISTRATION OF LIQUID MEDICATION

Procedure

Technical Action	Rationale/Amplification
1. Check medication to be administered, using "The Five Rights": right patient, right drug, right dose, right route, right time and frequency.	1. It is important to take measures to prevent errors of medication administration.
2. Wash hands.	2. Washing hands between patients is important in controlling communicable diseases in a hospital. It is advisable to wear nonsterile examination gloves while administering oral medication to an animal with a communicable disease.

Technical Action

3. Place liquid medication in syringe or small bottle.

4. With one hand, form a pouch from animal's cheek just caudal to commissures of its lips by placing finger or thumb inside cheek and pulling laterally on the lip (Fig. 5-3).

5. Place liquid medication into cheek pouch, small amounts at a time (Fig. 5-4).

6. Give medication slowly.

Rationale/Amplification

3. A spoon may be used to administer palatable liquids to animals of quiet temperament.

4. The animal's jaws therefore can remain closed during the procedure.

5. The dorsal surface of the animal's snout should be parallel to the ground or only slightly elevated while liquids are administered. Avoiding pointing the animal's nostrils toward the ceiling minimizes the possibility of aspiration of the liquid into the respiratory tract.

6. To ensure adequate dosing, it is advisable to administer a small amount of liquid and wait until the animal swallows before placing any more liquid into the cheek pouch.

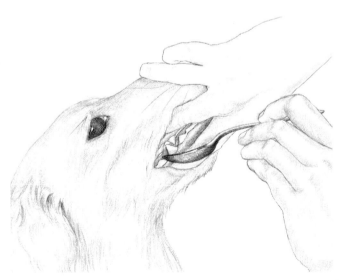

Figure 5-3 Forming a cheek pouch for administration of liquids.

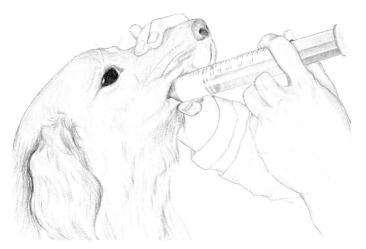

Figure 5-4   Administering liquid medication orally.

Technical Action

7. Note in animal's medical record that medication was given.

Rationale/Amplification

7. The following information should be noted in the medical record: date, time, medication, dosage, route, initials of individual administering medication, and comments.

Bibliography

Giving Medications, A Nursing Photobook. In Nursing '80 Photobook. Springhouse, PA, Intermed Communications, 1980

Jones BV: Animal Nursing, Part 2. Oxford, Pergamon Press, 1966

Kirk RW, and Bistner SI: Handbook of Veterinary Procedures and Emergency Treatment, 4th ed. Philadelphia, WB Saunders, 1985

McCurnin DM: Clinical Textbook for Veterinary Technicians. Philadelphia, WB Saunders, 1985

Chapter 6

DERMATOLOGIC PROCEDURES

What we see depends mainly on what we look for.

JOHN LUBBOCK

This chapter describes several procedures that are useful for gathering diagnostic information about skin diseases.

SKIN CULTURE

Skin culture is the inoculation of suitable media with material from the skin.

Purposes

1. To identify bacterial and fungal pathogens of the skin
2. To determine the antibiotic sensitivity of bacterial skin pathogens

Equipment Needed

- Cotton
- Culture media
- Sterile 22-gauge needle or scalpel blade (for bacterial culture)
- Scalpel blade or hemostatic forceps (for fungal culture)
- 70% alcohol (for bacterial culture)

Restraint and Positioning

An assistant restrains the animal in a position that affords access to the skin lesion(s) (see Chap. 1).

Bacterial Culture of a Skin Pustule

Procedure

Technical Action

1. Clip hair in square-inch area around pustule.
2. Cleanse clipped area gently with cotton moistened with 70% alcohol.

3. Let the skin air dry.

4. Insert tip of swab into pustule after puncturing it with sterile 22-gauge needle or after incising the pustule with point of No. 11 scalpel blade.
5. Inoculate material into suitable bacterial culture media.

6. Cleanse open pustule with 70% alcohol.

Rationale/Amplification

1. Clipping must be done carefully to avoid rupturing the pustule.
2. Disinfection of the pustule with 70% alcohol removes surface contaminants that might invalidate the culture results.
3. Do not collect material while skin is still moist because excess alcohol may be transferred to the swab.

5. The culture media can be inoculated directly, or the swab can be placed in transport medium.

Culture for Dermatophytes

Procedure

Technical Action

1. Cleanse edge of lesion with cotton moistened with water.

2. Using scalpel blade or hemostat, scrape or pluck several hairs from edge of lesion.

3. Inoculate dermatophyte culture medium with hairs by forcing hairs below the surface of medium.
4. Place cover on culture medium but do not close tightly.

Rationale/Amplification

1. Gentle cleansing with water removes superficial debris but will not interfere with fungal culture results.
2. Recovery of dermatophytes is most successful if visibly diseased hairs from the edge of the lesion are cultured.
3. Forcing of hairs below the surface of the medium ensures contact of dermatophytes on the hair with the culture medium.
4. Fungal growth may be enhanced by placing the medium in the dark.

Technical Action	Rationale/Amplification
5. Incubate at room temperature and check daily for growth.	5. Dermatophyte organisms will cause a color change in dermatophyte test medium when minimal growth is visible.

SKIN SCRAPING

Skin scraping is a diagnostic procedure involving intentional abrasion of a skin lesion with a scalpel blade.

Purpose

To detect the presence of microscopic skin parasites

Complication

Minor hemorrhage

✳ Equipment Needed

- Scalpel blade
- Glass slides
- Mineral oil or potassium hydroxide

Restraint and Positioning

An assistant restrains the animal in a position that affords access to the skin lesion(s) (see Chap. 1).

Procedure

Technical Action	Rationale/Amplification
1. Place one drop of mineral oil on each of several glass slides.	
2. Insert edge of scalpel blade into mineral oil on glass slide.	2. Moistening the scalpel blade with mineral oil provides a sticky surface for collecting mites and ova during the scraping.
3. Select lesion(s) to be scraped, avoiding areas of severe excoriation.	3. If sarcoptic mange is suspected, lesions on the ears, elbows, and hocks should be scraped.

Technical Action

4. Pinch fold of skin and scrape surface until drops of capillary blood appear (Fig. 6-1).

5. Transfer hair and epithelial debris collected from skin scraping into drop of mineral oil on glass slide by swirling or scraping material on slide edge.

6. Examine immediately.

7. Note results of skin scrapings in animal's medical record.

Rationale/Amplification

4. Pinching the skin helps to move the demodectic mites out of the deeper parts of the hair follicles. The normally deep location of demodectic mites within the skin necessitates scraping to the level of capillaries.

5. Several scrapings should be made and the site of the scraping indicated on each glass slide. As many as 20 scrapings may be necessary to obtain sarcoptic mites.

6. If potassium hydroxide is used, waiting several minutes may result in some clearing of the prepared specimens.

7. Note date, scraping sites, number of live and dead mites, larvae, and ova at each site. This is especially important in following the progress of animals being treated with parasiticides.

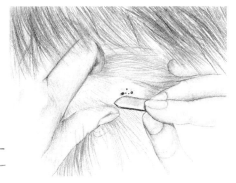

Figure 6-1 Skin scraping. Note that a fold of skin is pinched between the fingers to move mites out of hair follicles.

CELLOPHANE TAPE PREPARATION

A *cellophane tape preparation* is used to collect material from the surface of the skin and hair coat.

Purpose

To detect the presence of certain skin parasites, including flea larvae, lice, and mites. (Superficial skin mites)

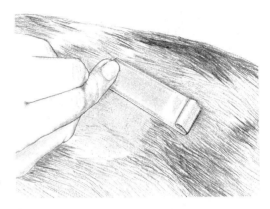

Figure 6-2 Collecting specimen from skin, using cellophane tape.

Equipment Needed

- Clear cellophane tape
- Glass slides
- Mineral oil

Restraint and Positioning

The animal is restrained in sternal recumbency or in a sitting or standing position.

Procedure

Technical Action

1. Select site for sampling.

2. Tear off a 1- to 2-inch piece of cellophane tape, attach one end to a glass slide, and double it back onto the slide so that sticky side does not contact slide.

3. Part hair and touch sticky side of clear cellophane tape to hair and skin (Fig. 6-2).

4. Place a drop of mineral oil on glass slide and flip tape so that sticky side with collected debris attaches to the slide and covers the oil.

Rationale/Amplification

1. Choose an area in which seborrhea or black debris is present, usually along the dorsal midline.

3. Loose particles will adhere to the tape. The attached slide adds rigidity to the tape and may improve collection of parasites.

Technical Action	Rationale/Amplification
5. Examine under microscope and note findings in animal's medical record.	**5.** Note date, sampling site, number, and identity of parasitic organisms collected.

SKIN BIOPSY

Skin biopsy is the removal of a small section of skin for histopathology or for making impression smears. A very small skin lesion may be excised completely by means of the biopsy procedure.

Purposes

1. To demonstrate the presence of bacterial, fungal, or parasitic organisms responsible for a particular skin disorder
2. To diagnose immune-mediated skin diseases
3. To identify skin neoplasms
4. To further characterize skin lesions for which fine-needle aspiration did not provide a definitive diagnosis.

Complications

1. Minor hemorrhage
2. Infection
3. Scar formation

Equipment Needed

- Clipper with No. 40 blade
- Skin preparation materials
    Cotton
    Mild soap (*not* povidone–iodine)
    70% alcohol
    Sterile gauze sponges (2″ × 2″)
- Sterile equipment for biopsy procedure
    Surgeon's gloves
    Surgical drape
    Gauze sponges (2″ × 2″)
    Fine-tooth forceps
    4-mm Keyes cutaneous biopsy punch* or No. 15 scalpel blade
    Needle-holding forceps
    Nonabsorbable suture material

*J. Sklar Manufacturing Co., Long Island City, NY.

- Equipment for local anesthesia
  - 1-ml syringe
  - 25-gauge needle
  - Local anesthetic solution (*e.g.,* 2% lidocaine)
- Materials for handling biopsy specimen
  - 25-gauge needle
  - Paper towels
  - Container with preservative: 10% formalin or 3% buffered glutaraldehyde (for electron microscopy)
  - Glass slides for impression smears
- Drugs for sedation (if necessary)

Restraint and Positioning

An assistant restrains the animal in a position that affords access to the skin lesion(s). It may be necessary to tranquilize or sedate uncooperative animals.

Preparation for Skin Biopsy

Procedure

Technical Action	Rationale/Amplification
1. Select appropriate biopsy site.	1. Avoid traumatized, crusted, or atypical lesions. Different stages of lesions, as well as normal tissue, should be biopsied. If possible, try to take a sample that includes the transition from normal to abnormal tissue.
2. Clip hair carefully from site.	2. It is important to avoid traumatizing the area to be biopsied during the clipping.
3. Prepare clipped area by washing gently with mild soap and applying 70% alcohol.	3. Vigorous scrubbing may distort the microscopic findings and therefore should be avoided. Iodine preparations should not be used because they can interfere with histologic staining.
4. Instill 0.5 ml to 1 ml of local anesthetic intradermally and subcutaneously around and beneath biopsy site.	4. Avoid instilling local anesthetic directly into the lesion to be biopsied because this may cause artifacts in the preparation.
5. Place surgical drape around biopsy site and don sterile gloves.	

Cutaneous Punch Biopsy

Procedure

Technical Action	Rationale/Amplification
1. Prepare for biopsy.	**1.** See p. 74.
2. Press skin biopsy punch firmly onto chosen site while applying rotary motion, until the entire skin has been penetrated (Fig. 6-3).	**2.** Use fingers of the other hand to stretch the skin over the biopsy site while the punch is introduced.
3. Remove punch from site and hold firm pressure on site with sterile gauze sponges to stop bleeding.	**3.** Hemostasis after biopsy is best achieved with firm pressure because cauterizing agents may enhance scar formation.
4. If necessary, use a 25-gauge needle to skewer biopsy core and raise it above the skin level. Cut base off with sharp scissors or scalpel blade (Fig. 6-4).	**4.** In many instances the biopsy core will remain *in situ* instead of being contained in the instrument lumen.
5. Carefully remove biopsy specimen from punch instrument with 20-gauge needle.	**5.** An additional specimen may be taken for the purpose of making impression smears.
6. Blot specimen on paper to remove excess blood.	**6.** See Chap. 7, pp. 78–80.
7. Make impression smears or place in container with preservative.	**7.** See Chap. 7, pp. 78–80.
8. Suture skin incision.	**8.** One or two single interrupted sutures usually are adequate to achieve primary closure.

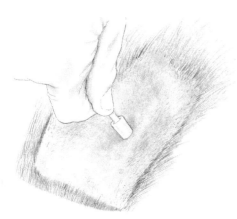

Figure 6-3 Using skin biopsy punch.

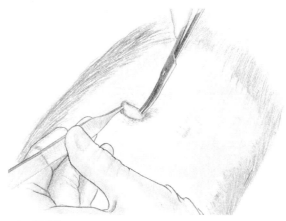

Figure 6-4 Severing base of biopsy specimen from underlying tissues.

Cutaneous Wedge Biopsy (Elliptical Incisional Biopsy)

Procedure

Technical Action

1. Select appropriate biopsy site and prepare for biopsy.

2. Make elliptical incision, extending from normal tissue into lesion through entire skin thickness.

3. Sever any subcutaneous attachments with sharp scissors, and remove wedge of tissue created by incision (Fig. 6-5).

4. Hold firm pressure on site with sterile gauze sponges to stop bleeding.

Rationale/Amplification

1. Avoid traumatized, crusted, or atypical lesions. Different stages of lesions, as well as normal tissue, should be biopsied. If possible, try to take a sample that includes the transition from normal to abnormal tissue. See p. 74, Nos. 1 to 5.

2. An incision 1 cm to 2 cm in length is usually sufficient for biopsy. A slightly longer incision may be necessary if the lesion is surrounded by fibrous tissue.

4. Hemostasis after biopsy is best achieved with firm pressure because cauterizing agents may enhance scar formation.

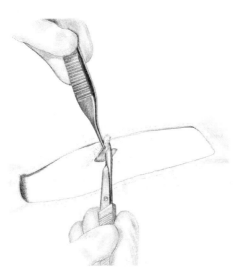

Figure 6-5 Removing cutaneous wedge by elliptical incisional biopsy.

Technical Action	**Rationale/Amplification**
5. Blot biopsy specimen with paper to remove excess blood.	**5.** See Chap. 7, pp. 78–80.
6. Make impression smears and place in container with preservative.	**6.** See Chap. 7, pp. 78–80.
7. Suture skin incision.	**7.** Simple interrupted, nonabsorbable sutures are appropriate for most biopsy sites.

Bibliography

Allen SK, McKeever PJ: Skin biopsy techniques. Vet Clin North Am 4(2): 269–280, 1974

Kirk RW, Bistner SI: Handbook of Veterinary Procedures and Emergency Treatment, 4th ed. Philadelphia, WB Saunders, 1985

Muller GH, Kirk RW: Small Animal Dermatology, 2nd ed. Philadelphia, WB Saunders, 1976

Stannard AA: Current concepts in small animal dermatology. 59th Annual Postgraduate Conference for Veterinarians, Michigan State University, East Lansing, MI, January 27, 1982

Chapter 7

IMPRESSION PREPARATIONS

Aim for perfection. Half right is always half wrong.

LAWRENCE LEVESON

Impression preparations (smears) are samples for cytologic evaluation, obtained by imprinting removed masses, biopsy specimens, or masses *in situ* onto microscope slides. Specimens that can be used for impression smears include ulcerated tumors, surgically excised tumors, and core biopsy specimens.

Purposes

1. To differentiate among causes of organomegaly involving lymph nodes, spleen, kidneys, liver, prostate, mammary glands, and other organs
2. To differentiate among inflammation, hyperplasia, and neoplasia as the cause of skin, subcutaneous, and other accessible tumors
3. To differentiate benign from malignant neoplasms, for diagnostic and therapeutic planning purposes
4. To differentiate carcinomas from sarcomas, for diagnostic and therapeutic planning purposes

Equipment Needed

- Scalpel blade
- Glass slides
- Sterile gauze
- Paper towel or blotter

Procedure

Technical Action

1. Prepare specimen in the following manner:

   Excised mass—incise mass with sharp scalpel blade, then blot until dry.

   Biopsy sample—blot specimen repeatedly until no visible fluid soils paper (Fig. 7-1).

   Mass *in situ*—clean surface by scraping with sterile gauze or scalpel blade. Blot mass repeatedly.

2. Touch biopsy or mass lightly to a clean glass slide and withdraw immediately. Make several imprints on each slide (Fig. 7-2).

Rationale/Amplification

1. To ensure adequate cellular material for interpretation, a freshly cut surface free of contamination by blood and exudate is needed. Care should be taken not to crush the specimen.

2. Firm pressure is not required. If exfoliation does not occur, the specimen may be lightly scraped.

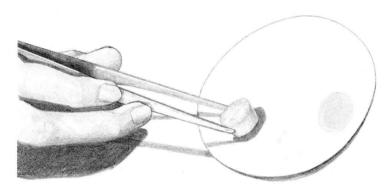

Figure 7-1   Blotting tissue specimen on paper until dry.

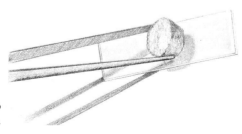

Figure 7-2   Touching tissue specimen to glass slide to make impression preparation.

Technical Action	Rationale/Amplification
3. Make several slides.	**3.** Having several slides allows the cytologist to use multiple stains, if necessary for diagnosis.

Bibliography

Allen SK, McKeever PJ: Skin biopsy techniques. Vet Clin N Am 4: 269–280, 1974

Perman V, Alsaker RD, Riis RC: Cytology of the Dog and Cat, pp. 1–5. South Bend Indiana, American Animal Hospital Association Monograph, 1979

Rebar AH: Handbook of Veterinary Cytology. St Louis, Purina Company Monograph, 1981

Stevens JB, Perman V, Osborne CA: Biopsy sample management, staining, and examination. Vet Clin North Am 4: 233–253, 1974

Chapter 8

FINE-NEEDLE ASPIRATION BIOPSY

Not failure, but low aim, is a crime.

LOWELL

— you must get into the cells you want.

Fine-needle aspiration biopsy is a diagnostic procedure involving introduction of a narrow-gauge, rigid hypodermic needle into a tissue or organ and removal of a small amount of tissue by suction. *V. commonly used (for any tissue in body) * get a good sample (representative)*

Purposes

1. To differentiate among causes of organomegaly involving lymph nodes, spleen, mammary glands, and other organs
2. To differentiate among inflammation, hyperplasia, and neoplasia as the cause of skin, subcutaneous, and other accessible tumors *pre-cancer new growth*
3. To differentiate benign from malignant neoplasms, for diagnostic and therapeutic planning purposes
4. To differentiate carcinomas from sarcomas, for diagnostic and therapeutic planning purposes
5. *Help to gain more info.*

Complications

1. Minor hemorrhage *at a superficial level ; puncturing another organ*
2. Tissue damage
3. *shooting-in-the-Dark (Not knowing if you're in the right place)*

Equipment Needed

- 22- to 25-gauge, 3/4″ to 3 1/2″ sterile needles
- 3-ml syringe
- Glass slides

ANIMAL MUST BE STILL → gen. anesthesia

Procedure

Technical Action

1. With animal restrained in an appropriate position, isolate lesion in one hand.
2. Prepare skin overlying lesion.

3. Carefully introduce needle, with syringe tightly attached, into lesion.

4. Apply negative pressure at needle bevel end by withdrawing syringe plunger (Fig. 8-1).

Rationale/Amplification

1. Local or general anesthesia is not required, except in rare instances.
2. For most lesions, simple cleansing and disinfection of the skin is all that is required. Intracavitary tumors or heavily soiled areas should have the hair clipped and the skin carefully scrubbed and disinfected.
3. In large lesions, the needle is directed into the peripheral parts of the lesion to avoid the necrotic center.
4. Several brisk excursions of the syringe plunger are made.

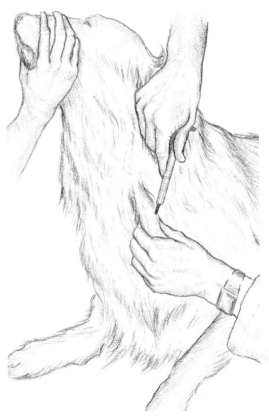

Figure 8-1 Aspiration of lymph node or other mass by brisk withdrawal of syringe plunger, creating suction at needle bevel.

Technical Action

5. Partially withdraw needle and redirect it into lesion (Fig. 8-2).
6. Again apply suction by several brisk movements of syringe plunger.
7. Release negative pressure by allowing syringe plunger to retract, and withdraw needle from lesion.
8. Separate needle from syringe and draw air into syringe.
9. Reattach syringe to needle and expel contents of needle lumen onto clean microscope slides (Fig. 8-3).

Rationale/Amplification

5. This step helps to ensure adequate sampling of the lesion.

7. Release of the negative pressure retains the sample within the needle lumen.

9. Expulsion should be rapid and forceful to remove all material from the needle lumen. Only a small drop of fluid is obtained in most aspirations.

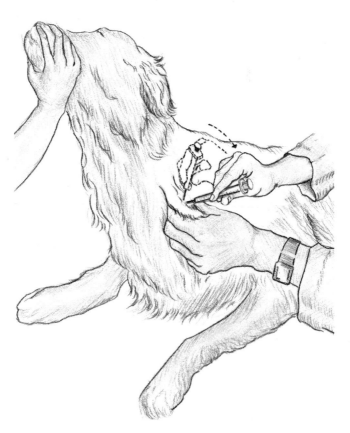

Figure 8-2 Partial withdrawal and redirection of needle/syringe assembly.

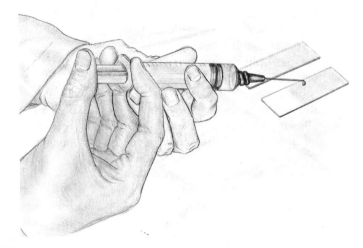

Figure 8-3 Expelling aspirated fluid from needle lumen with air-filled syringe.

Technical Action

10. Make smears of aspirated fluid immediately.

Rationale/Amplification

10. Push smears or squash preparations are made, depending on fluid viscosity. Squash preparations are more successful in producing thin smears when the fluid is highly viscous. Smears may be stained with a variety of stains. Whenever possible, three or four slides should be made.

Bibliography

Rebar AH: Handbook of Veterinary Cytology. St Louis, Purina Company, 1981

Soderstrom N: Fine-Needle Aspiration Biopsy. New York, Grune & Stratton, 1966

Chapter 9

OPHTHALMIC PROCEDURES

If a blind man guides a blind man, both will fall into a pit.

MATTHEW 15:14

※ OCCLUDED TEAR DUCT

This chapter describes a number of diagnostic and therapeutic procedures that are commonly used in caring for the eye.

Diagnostic Procedures

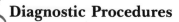

- Schirmer tear test
- Corneoconjunctival culture
- Staining of the cornea
- Corneoconjunctival smear and scraping
- Schiotz tonometry

NOTE: *These procedures are listed in an order conducive to proceeding from one procedure to the next. For proper management and use of the procedures, consideration of the animal's signs and careful planning of the appropriate sequence is recommended. See rationale/amplification comments in each section.*

Therapeutic Procedures

- Topical administration of ophthalmic medication
- Subconjunctival injection
- Flushing of nasolacrimal duct

Restraint and Positioning

An assistant restrains the animal in sternal recumbency or in a sitting position for most of the procedures. Topical administration of ophthalmic medication usually can be accomplished without the aid of an assistant. If the animal is fractious, it will be necessary to apply a muzzle or to tranquilize the animal.

SCHIRMER TEAR TEST

Purpose

To assess the amount of tear production in each eye

Complications

1. Corneal irritation
2. Corneoconjunctival infection

Equipment Needed

- Schirmer tear test strips*
- Metric ruler
- Topical ophthalmic anesthetic

Procedure

Technical Action

1. Perform Schirmer tear test I before any other procedures on eye.

2. While keeping test strip within sterile package, fold strip at notch.

3. Remove sterile strip from package and insert folded end between lower eyelid and cornea near lateral canthus (Fig. 9-1).

Rationale/Amplification

1. The results of the test will be affected by other procedures involving eyelid manipulations, instillation of topical materials, and procurement of specimens.

2. The notched end of the strip should be kept sterile because this is the portion that will be placed in contact with the eye.

3. Avoid moving the strip across the cornea. In the Schirmer tear test I, the rate of basal and reflex tear production is measured as the animal tears in response to the sensation of the strip contacting the eye.

*SMP Division, Cooper Laboratories, Inc., San German, PR 00753.

Technical Action

4. Hold strip in place for 1 minute and prevent the animal from rubbing the eye.

5. Remove strip and measure length of strip from notch to wet/dry interface according to package instructions.

6. To perform Schirmer tear test II
   a. Lift upper eyelid with index finger and instill one to two drops of topical ophthalmic anesthetic at 12 o'clock position on globe (Fig. 9-2).
   b. Wait 30 to 60 seconds. *tear stains strip*
   c. Prevent animal from rubbing its eye.

7. Repeat Nos. 2 to 5 as for Schirmer tear test I.

Rationale/Amplification

strip will absorb tears

5. The normal rate of basal and reflex tear production, as measured by the Schirmer tear test I, in cats and dogs is 13 to 25 mm/min. (NORMAL)

6. Specimens for bacteriologic cultures should be obtained before conducting Schirmer tear test II because topical solutions can interfere with culture results.

7. The Schirmer tear test II performed under topical anesthesia measures the basal tear flow. The value obtained should be approximately one half that of the Schirmer tear test I.

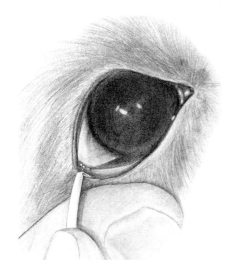

Figure 9-1 Schirmer tear test strip in place between lower eyelid and cornea.

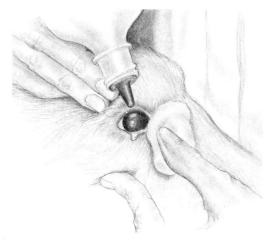

Figure 9-2 Instilling topical ophthalmic anesthetic. Note that the drops are placed at the 12 o'clock position on the globe.

CORNEOCONJUNCTIVAL CULTURE

Purposes

1. To identify bacterial, fungal, and other pathogens of the cornea and conjunctiva, especially in severe, chronic, or nonresponsive conditions
2. To determine the antibiotic sensitivity of corneoconjunctival pathogens

Complication

Corneal irritation

Equipment Needed

- Sterile swabs for bacterial and fungal cultures
- Tube with transport medium
- Specific bacterial and fungal culture media (if desired)

Procedure

Technical Action

1. Obtain specimens for culture before instilling any topical ophthalmic medications.
2. Moisten end of culture swab with liquid transport medium.

3. Evert lower eyelid by pulling downward on skin just below lower eyelid margin with index finger.
4. Gently swab cornea and conjunctival sac, avoiding eyelid margins (Fig. 9-3).
5. Replace swab in transport tube or inoculate culture media immediately.

Rationale/Amplification

1. Topical medications, including anesthetics, can interfere with culture results.
2. There is better recovery of organisms and less chance of corneal irritation if a moistened swab is used to obtain the specimen.
3. Do not put finger in palpebral fissure.

4. Debris and normal skin flora on eyelid margins can interfere with the accuracy of culture results.
5. Transport inoculated media to laboratory as soon as possible.

STAINING OF THE CORNEA

Purposes

1. To determine presence, location, and severity of corneal ulcers
2. To demonstrate patency of nasolacrimal duct

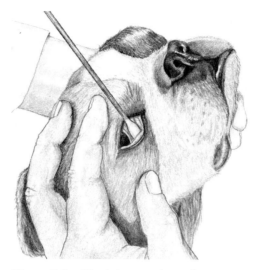

Figure 9-3 Obtaining specimen for corneo-conjunctival culture.

Equipment Needed

• Ophthalmic irrigating solution (*e.g.* Dacriose*)
• Sterile fluorescein impregnated strips† or fluorescein ophthalmic solution

Procedure

Technical Action

1. Perform corneal staining after Schirmer tear test I and after specimens have been obtained for bacteriologic culture and cytology but before instilling topical ophthalmic anesthetic.

2. Moisten end of sterile fluorescein strip‡ with ophthalmic irrigating solution or artificial tear solution. *(or Saline)*

3. Elevate upper eyelid and place moistened tip of fluorescein strip against bulbar conjunctiva for one or two seconds (Fig. 9-4).

4. Remove strip and allow animal to blink.

Rationale/Amplification

1. The stain will interfere with the results of these tests. Use of a topical ophthalmic anesthetic may result in a false-positive stain reaction.

2. The sterile fluorescein strips are recommended over the fluorescein solution because the solution can easily become contaminated with microorganisms.

3. It is important to avoid touching the fluorescein strip directly to the cornea because this may cause staining artifacts.

4. Blinking helps to distribute the stain.

*SMP Division, Cooper Laboratories, Inc., San German, PR 00753
†Fluor-I-Strip, Ayerst Laboratories, Inc., New York, NY 10017.

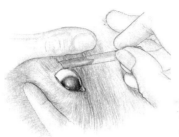

Figure 9-4 Staining of cornea with fluorescein. Note that fluorescein strip is applied to the bulbar conjunctiva rather than directly to the cornea.

Technical Action

5. Liberally flush eye with ophthalmic irrigating solution.
6. Examine cornea in a partially darkened room.

7. Observe external nares for emergence of green dye.

Rationale/Amplification

5. The sodium ions in the solution will enhance the stain.
6. The exposed corneal stroma in an ulcer stains bright green with fluorescein. Use of an ultraviolet light source (*i.e.* Wood's lamp) may enhance the observer's perception of stromal stain retention.
7. The appearance of fluorescein dye at the nostril indicates patency of the nasolacrimal duct.

CORNEOCONJUNCTIVAL SMEAR AND SCRAPING

Purpose

To obtain specimen(s) for cytologic examination

Complication

Corneal irritation

Equipment Needed

- Topical ophthalmic anesthetic
- Glass slides
- Stains (one or more may be selected)
  Gram's stain
  Modified Giemsa stain
    2 ml of Wolbach modified Giemsa tissue stain*
    2 ml of Wright's buffer (pH 6.8)
    50 ml of distilled water
  New methylene blue stain

*Giemsa Tissue Stain, Wolbach Modification, Dade (Harleco), Division American Hospital Supply Corp., Gibbstown, NJ 08027.

- Sterile cotton swabs for smear
- Sterile metal ocular spatula for scraping

Procedure

Technical Action	**Rationale/Amplification**
1. Remove mucus or exudate from eyelids (Fig. 9-5).	1. Cleanse eyelids gently with water-moistened cotton balls so that excess debris is not collected inadvertently with the specimen.
2. Lift upper eyelid with index finger to expose sclera and instill one or two drops of topical ophthalmic anesthetic at 12 o'clock position on globe.	2. It is important that the anesthetic flow down over the entire cornea for adequate desensitization to occur.
3. Wait 30 to 60 seconds.	
4. Evert lower eyelid by pulling downward on skin just below lower eyelid margin.	
5. For smear preparation, swab cornea and conjunctiva with cotton-tipped applicator, avoiding eyelid margins (Fig. 9-3, p. 89). For scraping, gently rub area of cornea or conjunctiva with metal ocular spatula until a small droplet of material is collected (Fig. 9-6).	5. Debris and normal skin flora on eyelid margins can interfere with the accuracy of cytologic examination.

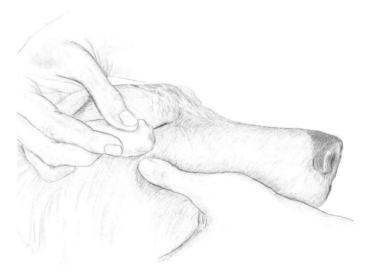

Figure 9-5   Removing mucus or exudate from eyelids.

Technical Action

6. Roll material from swab onto clean glass slides (Fig. 9-7). Spread material from scraping over glass slides.
7. Allow slides to air dry and then stain.

Rationale/Amplification

7. A gram-stained slide can be examined for bacteria. The modified Giemsa stain is useful for cytologic examination.

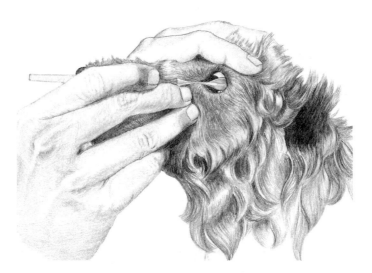

Figure 9-6 Obtaining corneoconjunctival scraping.

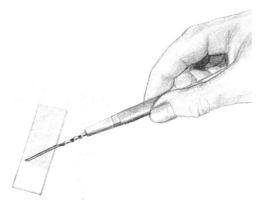

Figure 9-7 Placing corneoconjunctival specimen on glass slide.

Technical Action	Rationale/Amplification
8. For Giemsa staining: Fix slide for 5 minutes in absolute methanol; stain with modified Giemsa stain for 20 minutes; rinse with running tap water, and allow to air dry.	
9. Prevent animal from rubbing its eye.	**9.** Instillation of topical medication often is followed by the animal attempting to rub its eye.

SCHIOTZ TONOMETRY

※ Purpose

To measure intraocular pressure

Complication

Corneal irritation or erosion

Equipment Needed

- Topical ophthalmic anesthetic
- ✳ Schiotz's tonometer *keep dust free*

Procedure

Technical Action	Rationale/Amplification
1. Check tonometer before using.	**1.** Tonometer must be clean to ensure free movement of the plunger and to prevent contamination of the animal's cornea.
✳ *The animal must be calm (tranquilize)*	
2. Lift upper eyelid to expose sclera and instill one or two drops of topical ophthalmic anesthetic at 12 o'clock position on globe. *deader eye*	**2.** It is important that the anesthetic flow down over the entire cornea for adequate desensitization to occur.
3. Wait 30 to 60 seconds.	
4. Tilt animal's snout upward toward ceiling and retract lower eyelid with finger of one hand. *personal preference*	✳ **4.** Avoid applying pressure to the globe.

Technical Action

5. With other hand, grasp tonometer with thumb and index finger while resting other fingers on animal's skull just above upper eyelid. *Gently*
6. Place footplate of tonometer gently on central part of cornea such that tonometer is perpendicular to the cornea and to the floor (Fig. 9-8).

7. Note scale reading and remove tonometer.

Rationale/Amplification

5. Resting the hand holding the tonometer on the animal's head helps to steady it during the procedure.

6. Slide the holding sleeve bracket downward so that the entire weight of the tonometer rests on the cornea. Pressure on the jugular vein or excessive pressure on the eye will falsely elevate the tonometry results.
7. In general, the lower the reading on the tonometer instrument scale, the higher the intraocular pressure.

– only take 1 reading per time.

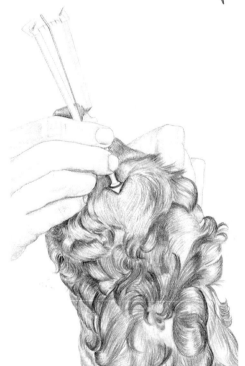

Figure 9-8 Placing Schiotz tonometer on cornea. *(Cataract surgery)*

✳ measure occular press.

Technical Action	Rationale/Amplification
8. If scale reading is 0 to 2, add weight and take another reading.	**8.** Readings are most accurate if taken with sufficient weight to allow the needle to rest in a middle scale position.
9. Repeat procedure two more times.	**9.** The scale readings can then be averaged. There should be a difference of no more than one unit between the three readings.
10. Record scale reading/tonometer weight and convert scale reading to mm Hg of intraocular pressure (IOP) by using table calibrated for canine eye.	**10.** The table used for human intraocular pressure (IOP) will give a lower than actual result for dogs. Normal IOP values in dogs and cats are 15 to 25 mm Hg.
11. Clean tonometer thoroughly after use, disassemble, and enclose in container.	**11.** The tonometer may be cleaned with ether. Pipe cleaners are useful for cleaning this instrument. Ultraviolet sterilizers are available.
12. Prevent animal from rubbing its eye.	**12.** Instillation of topical medication often is followed by attempts to rub eye.

TOPICAL ADMINISTRATION OF OPHTHALMIC MEDICATION

Purpose

To medicate cornea, conjunctiva, and anterior uveal tract

Complication

Self-trauma to the eye by the animal

Equipment Needed

- Ophthalmic irrigating solution (*e.g.,* Dacriose*)
- Cotton
- Ophthalmic solution or ointment
- Bandaging materials for paws (if necessary)
    Gauze
    Adhesive tape, 1 inch or 2 inches in width
- Elizabethan collar (if necessary)

*SMP Division, Cooper Laboratories, Inc., San German, PR 00753

Procedure

Technical Action

1. Cleanse eyelids and adjacent facial skin with cotton moistened with warm water.
2. Remove debris on cornea and conjunctival sac by everting eyelids and flushing thoroughly with ophthalmic irrigating solution.
3. Hold solution or ointment container between thumb and index finger of one hand while using third finger or heel of hand to lift upper eyelid.
4. Instill one or two drops of solution or small ribbon of ointment on sclera at 12 o'clock position on globe (Fig. 9-9). Then release eyelid.
5. If instilling several medications, wait at least 1 minute between applications, and always instill solutions before ointments.

6. Apply petroleum-based ointment to facial skin adjacent to eye if ocular discharge is present.

Rationale/Amplification

1. Keep animal's lids closed during cleansing to prevent trauma to cornea.
2. The eye and eyelids should be cleaned well before instilling medication to ensure effectiveness of treatment.

4. It is important to avoid contaminating the medicine bottle or tube by touching it to the eye or eyelids.

5. Solutions cannot readily penetrate a film of ointment. Topical medications will enter the nasolacrimal duct and therefore may be licked from the nose. Atropine has a bitter taste and may induce salivation.

6. The petroleum-based ointment will prevent scalding of the skin by the ocular discharges.

Put in drops before any ointments (sol.)

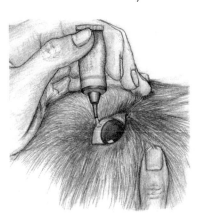

Figure 9-9 Instilling ophthalmic ointment.

Technical Action	Rationale/Amplification
7. Note in animal's medical record that medication was given.	**7.** Note date, time, medication, eye(s) medicated, comments and initials.
8. Prevent self-trauma to eye by bandaging dewclaws or entire feet or by placing Elizabethan collar on animal.	**8.** Animals commonly try to rub the eyes after topical medications, particularly solutions, are instilled.

SUBCONJUNCTIVAL INJECTION

Purpose

To medicate the anterior uveal tract

Complications

1. Systemic overdosage
2. Penetration of the globe by needle

Equipment Needed

- Cotton
- Ophthalmic irrigating solution (*e.g.*, Dacriose*)
- Topical ophthalmic anesthetic
- 25-gauge needle
- Tuberculin syringe
- Ocular fixation forceps
- Magnifying loupe (if desired)

Procedure

Technical Action	Rationale/Amplification
1. Cleanse eyelids and cornea as previously described.	**1.** See p. 96, Nos. 1 and 2.
2. Lift upper eyelid to expose sclera and instill one or two drops of topical ophthalmic anesthetic at 12 o'clock position on globe.	**2.** It is important that the anesthetic flow down over the entire eye for adequate desensitization to occur.
3. Wait 30 to 60 seconds.	
4. Ask assistant to lift animal's upper eyelid.	

*SMP Division, Cooper Laboratories, Inc., San German, PR 00753

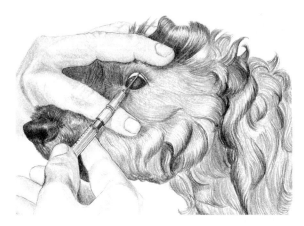

Figure 9-10 Performing subconjunctival injection.

Technical Action	**Rationale/Amplification**
5. Grasp bulbar conjunctiva with ocular fixation forceps and insert needle under bulbar conjunctiva (Fig. 9-10).	
6. Withdraw syringe plunger slightly. If no blood appears in syringe, inject medication. If blood appears in syringe, remove needle and select different site for injection.	6. No more than 0.25 ml should be injected at any one site.
7. Note in animal's medical record that medication was given.	7. Note date, time, medication, eye(s) medicated, comments, and initials.

FLUSHING OF NASOLACRIMAL DUCTS

Purposes

1. To determine patency of nasolacrimal duct
2. To relieve minor obstruction of nasolacrimal duct

Complication

Corneal irritation

Equipment Needed

- Cotton
- Ophthalmic irrigating solution (*e.g.,* Dacriose*)
- Topical ophthalmic anesthetic
- Sterile blunt metal probe (lacrimal duct dilator), 18- to 22-gauge
- Sterile cannula
- Syringe containing 5 ml sterile saline

Procedure

Technical Action	Rationale/Amplification
1. Cleanse eyelids and cornea as previously described.	1. See p. 96, Nos. 1 and 2.
2. Lift upper eyelid to expose sclera and instill one or two drops of topical ophthalmic anesthetic at 12 o'clock position on globe.	
3. Wait 30 to 60 seconds.	
4. Dilate upper and lower openings (puncta) of nasolacrimal duct with blunt metal probe of appropriate diameter (Fig. 9-11).	4. The puncta are located close to the medial canthus. Entering the opening is facilitated by slowly moving the metal probe along the inner lid margin toward the medial canthus while tensing the lid. The upper punctum is entered more easily than the lower.

*SMP Division, Cooper Laboratories, Inc., San German, PR 00753.

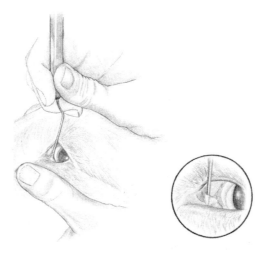

Figure 9-11 Dilating puncta of nasolacrimal duct with blunt metal probe.

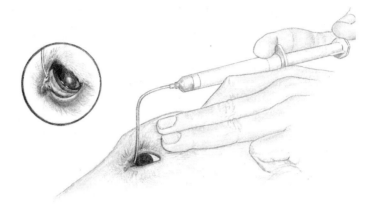

Figure 9-12 Flushing nasolacrimal duct.

Technical Action

5. Cannulate upper or lower punctum with commercial lacrimal cannula or with 20-gauge (or 22-gauge) plastic intravenous catheter (with needle removed).

6. Flush 3 to 5 ml sterile saline through cannulated punctum (Fig. 9-12).

7. See pp. 88–90 for use of fluorescein stain as an alternative method for determining patency of nasolacrimal duct.

Rationale/Amplification

5. Flushing of the duct can be accomplished by cannulating only one of the puncta.

6. If all of the flushing solution exits through the uncannulated punctum rather than at the nostril, try occluding the uncannulated punctum with finger tip or cotton swab.

7. The emergence of fluorescein at the external naris indicates the patency of the nasolacrimal duct.

Bibliography

Brightman AH: Current concepts in ocular pharmacology. Vet Clin North Am 10(2):261–280, 1980

Brunner LS, Suddarth DS: The Lippincott Manual of Nursing Practice, 3rd ed. Philadelphia, JB Lippincott, 1982

Glaze MB: Care of the ophthalmic patient. Compend Contin Educ for AHT 1(4):173–178, 1980

Magrane WC: Canine Ophthalmology, 3rd ed. Philadelphia, Lea & Febiger, 1977

Pratt PW (ed): Medical Nursing for Animal Health Technicians. Santa Barbara, CA, American Veterinary Publications, 1985

Severin GA: Veterinary Ophthalmology Notes, 2nd ed., Fort Collins, Colorado State University Press, 1979

Slatter DH: Fundamentals of Veterinary Ophthalmology. Philadelphia, WB Saunders, 1981

Whitley RD: Diagnostic and treatment techniques of corneal diseases in small animals. Compend Contin Educ for AHT 1(2):64–69, 1980

Chapter 10

EAR CARE

*Use what talents you possess: the woods would be very
silent if no birds sang there except those that sang best.*

HENRY VAN DYKE

Ear care includes cleaning and medicating of the external ear canal.

Purposes

1. To remove cerumen (waxy material) and other debris
2. To treat otitis externa
3. To prepare site for surgical procedures on the external ear canal

Complications

1. Rupture of tympanic membrane
2. Injury to external ear canal

Equipment Needed

- Cotton
- Bulb syringe or 10-ml hypodermic syringe
- Solution and waste bowls
- Cotton-tipped swabs
- Hemostat for hair removal (if necessary)
- Mild soap or ceruminolytic agents
- Otoscope
- Prescribed medication

Restraint and Positioning

Most tractable animals will tolerate ear cleaning and medicating with minimal restraint. An assistant holds the animal in sitting position or sternal recumbency, using one hand around the animal's snout to stabilize the animal's head. Fractious animals with painful ear infections may require general anesthetic or chemical tranquilization.

Procedure

Technical Action

1. Examine each ear carefully. Check for odor, ulceration, reddening, proliferation of tissue, discharge, or debris.

2. Examine each ear with otoscope starting with more normal ear (Fig. 10-1).

Rationale/Amplification

1. The external ear canal has a vertical portion leading to a horizontal portion that terminates at the tympanic membrane. It may be difficult to see the eardrum in older dogs. It is important to avoid contamination of a normal ear with debris from an infected ear.

2. Apply lateral tension to ear pinna (flap) to straighten ear canal as otoscope is advanced.

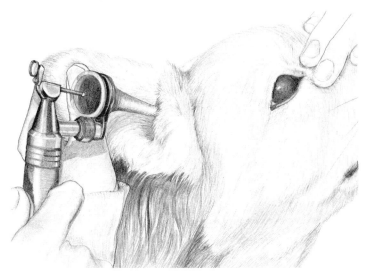

Figure 10-1 Examining ear with otoscope.

Technical Action

3. Remove hair if present, by grasping groups of hairs with hemostat and twisting handle of hemostat until hairs are gently removed (Fig. 10-2).

4. Instill ceruminolytic agent by dropper or mild soapy water by bulb syringe (Fig. 10-3), and gently massage skin over external ear canal.

5. Use pieces of cotton to remove loosened debris and discharge from ear canal (Fig. 10-4).

6. Repeat procedure as needed to remove all visible debris.

7. Rinse ear canal with warm water following procedures Nos. 4–6.

Rationale/Amplification

3. Poodles and some terriers normally have hair growing in their external ear canals. An alternative method of hair removal is simply to pluck the hairs out using fingers or a hemostat.

4. Excess irrigating solution can be caught in a waste bowl held beneath the ear. Massaging the skin over the external ear canal helps to loosen accumulated debris.

5. Cleansing of the ear canal with cotton wrapped around an index finger is a method that involves virtually no danger of rupturing the tympanic membrane.

6. Allowing the animal to shake its head from time to time will help dislodge debris in the deeper portions of the ear canal.

7. Residual soap or other cleansing agent may be irritating and can interfere with otic medication.

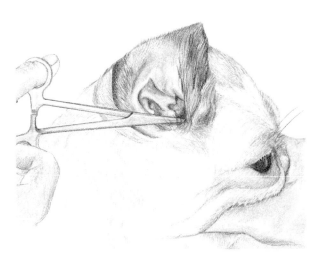

Figure 10-2 Removing hairs from external ear canal.

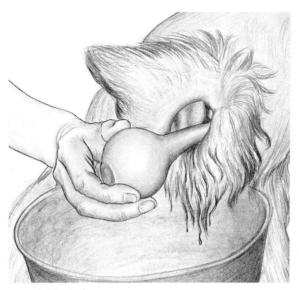

Figure 10-3 Instilling liquid agents into ear with bulb syringe.

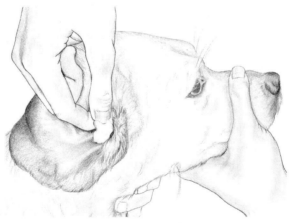

Figure 10-4 Removing loosened debris from ear canal with cotton.

Technical Action	**Rationale/Amplification**
8. Cleanse folds of skin on interior part of pinna with cotton-tipped swabs (Fig. 10-5).	8. Cotton-tipped swabs may be safely used on the ear flap but their use in the deeper portions of the ear canal is not recommended unless the animal is anesthetized.

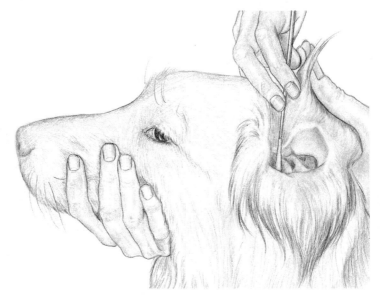

Figure 10-5 Cleansing interior folds of pinna with cotton-tipped swabs.

Technical Action	**Rationale/Amplification**
9. Dry ear canal as thoroughly as possible.	**9.** Use pieces of cotton and allow the animal to shake its head.
10. Inspect ear canal with otoscope.	**10.** Thoroughness of cleaning can be evaluated, and any lesions previously obscured by debris may be visible now.
11. Instill prescribed medication (drops or ointment) and massage external ear canal gently.	**11.** Massaging the ear aids in dispersal of the medication throughout the external ear canal. Note in animal's medical record date, time, medication, dosage, ear(s) medicated, initials, comments.

Bibliography

Brunner LS, Suddarth DS: The Lippincott Manual of Nursing Practice, 3rd ed. Philadelphia, JB Lippincott, 1982

Kirk RW, Bistner SI: Handbook of Veterinary Procedures and Emergency Treatment, 4th ed. Philadelphia, WB Saunders, 1985

McCurnin DM: Clinical Textbook for Veterinary Technicians. Philadelphia, WB Saunders, 1985

Chapter 11

PEDICURE

Small deeds done are better than great deeds planned.

PETER MARSHALL

Pedicure in cats and dogs consists of prophylactic or therapeutic trimming of the toenails.

Purposes

1. To prevent traumatic nail fracture
2. To trim or amputate damaged or ingrown toenails
3. To allow normal ambulation on footpads
4. To minimize physical damage to property, human beings, and other animals

Complications

1. Minor hemorrhage
2. Permanent deformity of toenails

Equipment Needed

- Commercial pet toenail clippers (guillotine type or scissors type)
- Cauterizing agent (*e.g.*, silver nitrate or ferric subsulfate applicators)

Restraint and Positioning

Nail trimming can be accomplished with the animal standing or in lateral recumbency. An assistant may be needed to restrain the animal. A muzzle or Elizabethan collar, and sometimes even chemical tranquilization, may be necessary if the animal objects to the procedure (see Chap. 1).

Procedure

Technical Action

1. If animal has light-colored toe-nails, note location of vascular matrix.

2. When using guillotine-type nail clippers

   a. Slide ring over nail and position clippers so that screws on clipper face the base of the toenail.
   b. Place ring 2 mm from end of vascular matrix.

   c. Clip nail by forcefully squeezing clipper handles together, thereby advancing the cutting blade (Fig. 11-1).

Rationale/Amplification

1. It is easy to avoid the pink matrix containing blood vessels and nerve supply if the animal has light-colored toenails.

2. This type of clipper is recommended for general use because it is inexpensive and can be used safely by pet owners for regular nail trimming.

   a. Holding the clippers in this way helps to prevent inadvertent clipping of the nail too short.
   b. If animal has dark-colored toenails, clip small amount of nail at a time and look at clipped cross-section. When the matrix is near the clipped edge, the cross-section will begin to appear "meaty" and lighter in color.

   c. The nail is severed by the beveled cutting blade as the latter slides across the rigid metal ring encircling the nail.

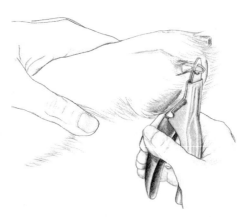

Figure 11-1 Clipping toenail using guillotine-type clippers.

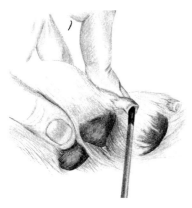

Figure 11-2 Cauterizing bleeding toenail matrix.

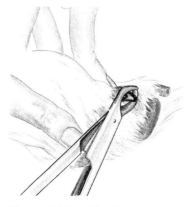

Figure 11-3 Clipping toenail using scissors-type clippers.

Technical Action	**Rationale/Amplification**
3. If bleeding from toenail occurs, apply cauterizing agent (Fig 11-2).	**3.** Silver nitrate-impregnated applicators or cotton swabs moistened with ferric subsulfate solution are effective cauterizing agents. Electrocautery can cause nail deformity and should not be used to stop hemorrhage from toenails, even if the animal is under general anesthesia.
4. Use scissors-type nail clippers for clipping toenails that have grown into foot pads (Fig. 11-3).	**4.** Ingrown toenails can result in painful inflammation or infection of the foot pad. Aftercare may include soaking the foot several times daily in warm epsom salt solutions.
5. Examine feet to make certain all toenails, including dewclaws, have been trimmed.	**5.** Regular monthly trimming or filing of toenails will cause the matrix to retract so that the nail length can gradually be shortened.

Bibliography

McCurnin DM: Clinical Textbook for Veterinary Technicians. Philadelphia, WB Saunders, 1985

Muller GH, Kirk RW: Small Animal Dermatology. Philadelphia, WB Saunders, 1969

Chapter 12

URETHRAL CATHETERIZATION

If at first you don't succeed, try, try, again. Then give up.
There's no use being a damn fool about it.

W.C. FIELDS

Urethral catheterization is the placement of a hollow device, a catheter, into the urethra.

Purposes

1. To collect urine for analysis or bacteriologic culture if the specimen cannot be obtained by percutaneous cystocentesis
2. To administer medication or radiographic contrast media directly into the urinary bladder.
3. To provide closed continuous drainage of urine (*e.g.,* when careful monitoring of urine output is necessary)
4. To relieve urethral obstruction

Complications

1. Trauma to urethra or urinary bladder
2. Urinary tract infection

Equipment Needed

1. For urethral catheterization of male dog
   - Cotton
   - Povidone–iodine surgical scrub

- Mild soap
- Sterile surgeon's gloves
- Sterile urinary catheter
- Sterile lubricating jelly
- Container for urine
- Tubing and antimicrobial ointment (if continuous urine drainage is to be established)

2. For urethral catheterization of female dog
   - Cotton
   - Povidone–iodine surgical scrub
   - Sterile surgeon's gloves
   - Sterile urinary catheter
   - Sterile lubricating jelly or antimicrobial ointment
   - 0.3 ml topical ophthalmic anesthetic or 0.5% lidocaine in tuberculin syringe with needle removed
   - Container for urine
   - Tubing and antimicrobial ointment (if continuous urine drainage is to be established)
   - Light source and sterile vaginal speculum for visual technique

3. For urethral catheterization of cat
   - Cotton
   - Povidone–iodine surgical scrub
   - Sterile surgeon's gloves
   - Sterile urinary catheter
   - Sterile lubricating jelly
   - Container for urine
   - Adhesive tape, 3–0 monofilament nonabsorbable suture material, tubing, antimicrobial ointment, and Elizabethan collar (if continuous urine drainage is to be established)
   - Drugs for tranquilization or anesthesia (if necessary)
   - 0.2 ml topical ophthalmic anesthetic or 0.5% lidocaine in tuberculin syringe, with needle removed (for female cat)

Restraint and Positioning

An assistant is needed to restrain the animal so that aseptic technique can be maintained throughout the procedure. The position preferred for urethral catheterization is lateral recumbency for the male dog, the male cat, and the female cat. Ideally, the female dog should be restrained in a standing position for urethral catheterization, but other acceptable positions are sternal or lateral recumbency.

PREPARATION FOR URETHRAL CATHETERIZATION

Procedure

Technical Action

1. Cleanse area around prepuce or vulva using povidone–iodine surgical scrub. Rinse thoroughly and dry.

2. Select catheter of appropriate size and type (see Table 12-1).

3. Wash hands thoroughly and don sterile surgeon's gloves.

Rationale/Amplification

1. It is advisable to clip long hairs from the area immediately surrounding the prepuce or vulva if continuous urine drainage is to be established.

2. To minimize trauma to the urinary tract, use the most flexible and the smallest diameter catheter that can be inserted easily. The Foley self-retaining catheter with an inflatable tip is available in sizes 8 and larger for continuous urine drainage.

3. Every precaution must be taken to reduce the chance of iatrogenic infection. Persons experienced in

TABLE 12-1. Recommended Urethral Catheter Sizes for Routine Use in Dogs and Cats

Animal	Catheter Type	Size*
Cat	Tomcat catheter (polyethylene)	3½ F
	Flexible vinyl or rubber urethral catheter	3½ F
Male dog (≤ 25 lb)	Polyethylene, vinyl, or rubber urethral catheter	3½ or 5 F
Male dog (> 25 lb)	Polyethylene, vinyl, or rubber urethral catheter	8 F
Male dog (> 75 lb)	Polyethylene, vinyl, or rubber urethral catheter	10 or 12 F
Female dog (≤ 10 lb)	Metal, polyethylene, vinyl, or rubber urethral catheter	5 F
Female dog (10 lb–50 lb)	Metal, polyethylene, vinyl, or rubber urethral catheter	8 F
Female dog (> 50 lb)	Metal, polyethylene, vinyl, or rubber urethral catheter	10, 12, or 14 F

* The diameter of urinary catheters is measured in French (F) units. One French unit equals ⅓ mm.

Technical Action	Rationale/Amplification
	urinary catheterization may be able to advance the catheter slowly out of its sterile package and thus maintain asepsis without wearing surgeon's gloves. Urethral catheterization requires two or more persons. It should not be attempted without assistance.
4. Examine catheter for flaws.	4. Discard any catheter that has a rough surface, eyes (holes) that are occluded, or a weakened area.

URETHRAL CATHETERIZATION OF MALE DOG

Procedure

Technical Action	Rationale/Amplification
1. Prepare for catheterization.	1. See pp. 112–113.
2. Estimate length of catheter needed to enter urinary bladder by holding catheter above dog in approximate position for catheterization (Fig. 12-1).	2. If a flexible catheter is advanced too far into the urinary bladder, the catheter can become knotted or folded back on itself within the bladder.

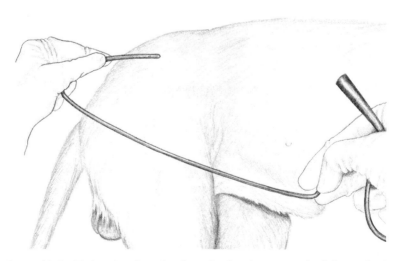

Figure 12-1   Estimating length of urethral catheter required for male dog.

Technical Action

3. *Assistant:* Place dog in lateral recumbency and abduct dog's upper rear leg. Then retract dog's prepuce such that distal 1 to 2 inches of glans penis is exposed (Fig. 12-2).

4. *Assistant:* Cleanse distal glans penis with mild soap.

5. *Operator:* Lubricate end of catheter liberally with sterile lubricating jelly and insert catheter tip into urethral orifice at distal end of glans penis (Fig. 12-3).

6 Advance catheter into urinary bladder.

7. If no urine appears when catheter has been advanced sufficiently to enter bladder, try to aspirate urine from catheter by a syringe.

Rationale/Amplification

3. To retract the prepuce, the assistant should apply pressure with the thumb at the point where the prepuce reflects onto the abdominal skin. The fingers of the hand can be placed gently around the penis but not so tightly as to constrict the urethra.

4. Any preputial glandular secretions are thereby removed.

5. In addition to facilitating passage, thorough lubrication of catheters reduces the chance of forcing bacteria from the distal urethra into the bladder. To prevent contamination of the catheter as it is being advanced, retain rest of catheter within sterile package or coiled within gloved hand.

6. Slight resistance may be encountered as the catheter passes over the ischial arch.

7. Advance catheter 1 inch to 2 inches farther if necessary. Manual compression of the urinary bladder to start urine flow is not recommended because this increases the risk of iatrogenic infection.

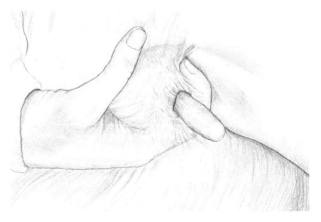

Figure 12-2 Retracting dog's prepuce.

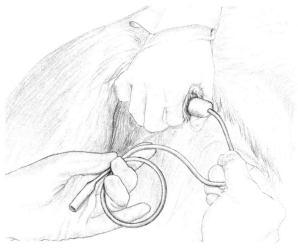

Figure 12-3 Inserting urethral catheter into penile urethra.

Technical Action

8. Collect urine specimen. (See pp. 124–126 for management of continuous urine drainage system.)

9. Withdraw catheter, using gentle traction, and note in animal's medical record that catheterization was performed.

Rationale/Amplification

8. We do not advise instilling dilute antiseptic solutions into the bladder after routine catheterization. Stock solutions of antiseptics may be contaminated with resistant bacteria.

9. Note date, time, catheter type and size, amount of urine collected, any medication instilled, comments, and initials.

URETHRAL CATHETERIZATION OF FEMALE DOG (VISUAL TECHNIQUE)

Procedure

Technical Action

1. Prepare for catheterization.
2. *Assistant:* Restrain dog in standing position and hold dog's tail to side (Fig. 12-4).

Rationale/Amplification

1. See pp. 112–113.
2. If dog's tail is held straight up, some dogs will strain or defecate during the procedure.

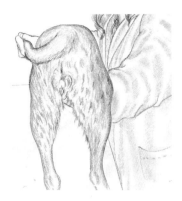

Figure 12-4 Restraint of female dog for urethral catheterization.

Technical Action

3. *Operator:* Insert lubricated sterile tuberculin syringe (with needle removed) containing 0.3 ml topical ophthalmic anesthetic or 0.5% lidocaine approximately 1½ inch to 2 inches into vagina and instill anesthetic.

4. Lubricate vaginal speculum and end of catheter liberally with sterile lubricating jelly.

5. Insert speculum into vagina with tip of speculum directed first dorsally, then cranially, to avoid clitoral fossa.

6. *Assistant:* Hold and adjust light source as necessary.

7. *Operator:* Introduce catheter through speculum into urethral orifice and advance into urinary bladder (Fig. 12-5).

Rationale/Amplification

3. Instillation of topical anesthetic will decrease the dog's discomfort and thus lessen struggling during the procedure.

4. For the visual technique, the catheter most easily introduced is either the rigid metal type or a Foley catheter equipped with a metal stylet.

5. The clitoral fossa is a blind sac just inside the ventral opening of the vulva. In addition to the usual vaginal speculum, a variety of instruments can be used to locate the urethral opening: laryngoscope, otoscope, modified empty syringe case, modified test tube.

6. The urethral orifice is located on the ventral surface of the vagina, approximately 1½ inch to 2 inches cranial to the opening of the vulva.

7. The urethra of the female dog is approximately 3 inches to 5 inches in length.

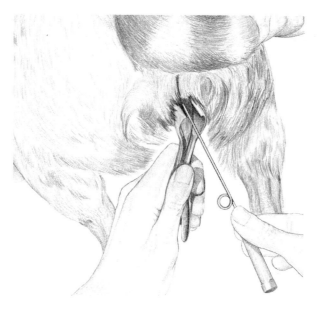

Figure 12-5 Introducing metal urethral catheter into female dog by visual technique.

Technical Action

8. If no urine appears when catheter has been advanced sufficiently to enter bladder, try to aspirate urine from catheter by a syringe.

9. Collect urine specimen. (See pp. 124–126 for management of continuous urine drainage system.)

10. Remove catheter and note in animal's medical record that catheterization was performed.

Rationale/Amplification

8. Advance catheter 1 inch to 2 inches farther if necessary. Care must be taken if the dog struggles while a rigid metal catheter is in place because it could perforate the bladder wall. Manual compression of the urinary bladder to start urine flow is not recommended because this increases the risk of iatrogenic infection.

9. We do not advise instilling dilute antiseptic solutions into the bladder after routine catheterization. Stock solutions of antiseptics may be contaminated with resistant bacteria.

10. Note date, time, catheter type and size, amount of urine collected, any medication instilled, comments, and initials.

URETHRAL CATHETERIZATION OF FEMALE DOG (TACTILE TECHNIQUE)

Procedure

Technical Action

1. Prepare for catheterization.
2. *Assistant:* Restrain dog in standing position and hold dog's tail to side.
3. *Operator:* Insert lubricated sterile tuberculin syringe (with needle removed), containing 0.3 ml topical ophthalmic anesthetic or 0.5% lidocaine approximately 1½ to 2 inches into vagina and instill anesthetic.
4. Lubricate gloved index finger of one hand and tip of flexible urethral catheter with sterile lubricating jelly or antimicrobial ointment.
5. Palpate urethral papilla (tissue surrounding urethral orifice) with gloved index finger of one hand.
6. Pass urethral catheter ventral to gloved finger in vagina and use finger to guide catheter down into urethral orifice while protecting rest of catheter from contamination with palm of hand (Fig. 12-6).

Rationale/Amplification

1. See pp. 112–113.
2. If dog's tail is held straight up, some dogs will strain or defecate during this procedure.
3. Instillation of topical anesthetic will decrease the dog's discomfort and therefore lessen struggling during the procedure.
4. Theoretically, the use of an antimicrobial ointment as a lubricant could interfere with bacteriologic cultures. Right-handed persons should hold the catheter coiled in the right hand and use the left hand to palpate the urethral orifice.
5. The urethral papilla is a ¼ inch to ½ inch, round, firm or soft mass in the ventral midline of the vagina approximately 1½ inch to 2 inches from the vulvar opening. The papilla is usually beneath the tip of the index finger when the finger has been inserted into the vagina to the level of the second knuckle.
6. With practice, this procedure can be done as quickly as the visual method on any dog 15 lb or larger. The advantages are that it usually is tolerated better by dogs than is the speculum technique and that it permits easy placement of flexible catheters. Flexible catheters must be used for continuous urine drainage.

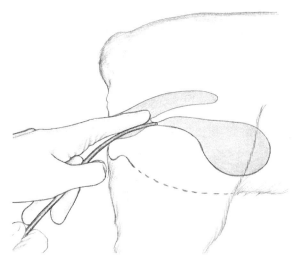

Figure 12-6 Introducing flexible urethral catheter into female dog by tactile technique.

Technical Action

7. If end of catheter can be palpated advancing past tip of index finger, withdraw catheter slightly and redirect it ventrally into urethral orifice.

8. Advance catheter into urinary bladder.

9. If no urine appears when catheter has been advanced sufficiently to enter bladder, try to aspirate urine from catheter by a syringe.

10. Collect urine specimen. (See pp. 124–126 for management of continuous urine drainage system.)

Rationale/Amplification

7. In such an instance, the catheter is probably being inserted into the proximal vagina toward the cervix.

8. The urethra of the female dog is approximately 3 to 5 inches in length, *i.e.,* it is relatively short as compared to that of the male dog.

9. Advance catheter 1 inch to 2 inches farther if necessary. Manual compression of the urinary bladder to start urine flow is not recommended because this increases the risk of iatrogenic infection.

10. We do not advise instilling dilute antiseptic solutions into the bladder after routine catheterization. Stock solutions of antiseptics may be contaminated with resistant bacteria.

Technical Action

11. Withdraw catheter by gentle traction and note in animal's medical record that catheterization was performed.

Rationale/Amplification

11. Note date, time, catheter type and size, amount of urine collected, any medication instilled, comments, and initials.

URETHRAL CATHETERIZATION OF MALE CAT

Procedure

Technical Action

1. Prepare for catheterization.

2. Tranquilize or anesthetize cat, if necessary.

3. *Assistant:* Restrain cat in lateral recumbency, grasp tail base, and deflect dorsally or laterally (Fig. 12-7).

4. Lubricate end of catheter with sterile jelly.

Rationale/Amplification

1. See pp. 112–113.

2. A person experienced in this procedure can perform it rapidly on a fully conscious, even-tempered cat.

3. An Elizabethan collar is a useful adjunct to restraint during this procedure.

4. A polyethylene tomcat catheter is most commonly used. A catheter with side holes and closed end is less traumatic to the urethra and bladder than is the open-ended type.

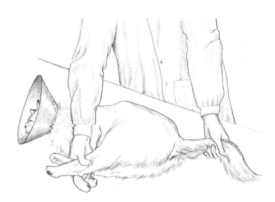

Figure 12-7 Restraint of male cat for urethral catheterization.

Technical Action

5. Place thumb and index finger of one hand on either side of prepuce so that palm of hand rests on cat's lower spine. Exert pressure with thumb and index finger in cranial direction to extrude penis from prepuce (Fig. 12-8).

6. Introduce catheter approximately ¾ inch into urethra such that holes in catheter tip are no longer visible (Fig. 12-9*A*).

7. Allow penis to retract within prepuce, leaving catheter in place.

8. Pinch preputial skin gently between thumb and forefinger and pull prepuce caudally and ventrally while advancing catheter into urinary bladder (Fig. 12-9*B*).

9. If catheter cannot be advanced because of urethral blockage, repeat procedure using 20-gauge 1-inch intravenous catheter (with needle removed) in place of urethral catheter. Flush catheter with sterile saline until urethral debris is dislodged.

Rationale/Amplification

5. The right-handed person should use the left hand to extrude the penis from the prepuce. If the penis is not adequately extruded from the prepuce (¾"–1"), catheterization will be very difficult.

8. Applying traction to the prepuce at this step straightens the flexure in the cat's penis and permits the catheter to pass over the ischial arch.

9. When the urethral blockage has been relieved, insert a tomcat catheter and empty bladder by aspirating urine by a syringe attached to the catheter. Manual compression should not be attempted if a bladder has been distended by an obstruction because perforation can result.

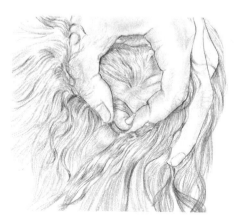

Figure 12-8 Extending cat's penis from prepuce.

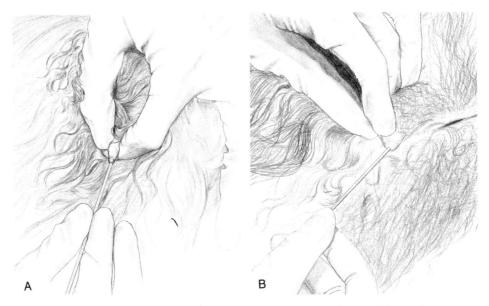

Figure 12-9 (*A*) and (*B*) Advancing urethral catheter into penile urethra.

Technical Action

10. Collect urine specimen. (See pp. 124–126 for management of continuous urine drainage system.)

11. Put Elizabethan collar on cat.

12. Remove catheter and note in animal's medical record that catheterization was performed.

Rationale/Amplification

10. Foley catheters are not available in sizes small enough for cats. If the catheter is to be left in place, adhesive tape is folded over the distal end of the catheter in a butterfly configuration. The "wings" of the tape are sutured once to the preputial skin on each side with nonabsorbable suture material.

11. Use of an Elizabethan collar will minimize the possibility of the cat deliberately removing the catheter.

12. Note date, time, catheter type and size, amount of urine collected, any medication instilled, comments, and initials.

URETHRAL CATHETERIZATION OF FEMALE CAT

Procedure

Technical Action

1. Prepare for catheterization.
2. *Assistant:* Restrain cat in lateral recumbency, grasp tail base, and deflect tail dorsally or laterally (See Fig. 12-7).
3. Tranquilize cat, if necessary, or insert lubricated sterile turberculin syringe (with needle removed) containing 0.2 ml topical ophthalmic anesthetic or 0.5% lidocaine approximately 1 inch into vagina and instill anesthetic.
4. Lubricate end of catheter liberally with sterile lubricating jelly.

5. Pull vulvar lips caudally while sliding catheter along ventral wall of vagina, until the catheter slips into the urethral orifice (Fig. 12-10).

Rationale/Amplification

1. See pp. 112–113.
2. An Elizabethan collar is a useful adjunct to restraint during this procedure.

3. Instillation of topical anesthetic will decrease the animal's discomfort and therefore lessen struggling during the procedure.

4. A 3½ F polyethylene tomcat catheter is a suitable urethral catheter for a female cat.
5. In many cases, the vagina of the female cat is too small to be opened with a speculum or for the tactile technique to be utilized. The "blind" technique can be successful if the operator is gentle and patient.

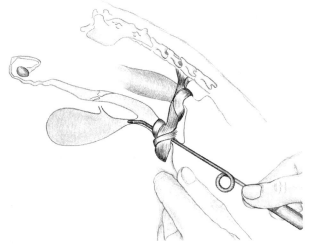

Figure 12-10 Introducing urethral catheter into female cat.

Technical Action	Rationale/Amplification
6. Collect urine specimen. (See pp. 124–126 for management of continuous urine drainage system.)	**6.** Foley catheters are not available in sizes small enough for cats. If the catheter is to be left in place, adhesive tape is folded over the distal end of the catheter in a butterfly configuration. The "wings" of the tape are sutured once to the perineal skin on each side with nonabsorbable suture material.
7. Put Elizabethan collar on cat.	**7.** Use of an Elizabethan collar will minimize the possibility of the cat deliberately removing the catheter.
8. Remove catheter and note in animal's medical record that catheterization was performed.	**8.** Note date, time, catheter type and size, amount of urine collected, any medication instilled, comments, and initials.

MANAGEMENT OF INDWELLING URETHRAL CATHETER AND CLOSED URINE DRAINAGE SYSTEM

Procedure

Technical Action	Rationale/Amplification
1. For continuous urine drainage, connect urethral catheter to collection container by means of sterile tubing (*e.g.,* intravenous fluid administration set).	**1.** Closed urine drainage carries less risk of urinary tract infection and prevents urine scalding of skin that can occur with an open indwelling urethral catheter.
2. Place collection container below level of animal's urinary bladder (Fig. 12-11).	**2.** Urine flow must be downhill to prevent backflow of contaminated urine into animal's bladder.
3. If Foley catheter is used: When catheter is draining well, inflate end of catheter according to manufacturer's directions.	**3.** Urethral trauma will occur if the inflatable portion has not been advanced into the urinary bladder when inflation is attempted.
4. Place Elizabethan collar on animal unless it is unconscious or can be observed constantly.	**4.** Animals can contaminate and remove urethral catheters, even if sutured to the skin.

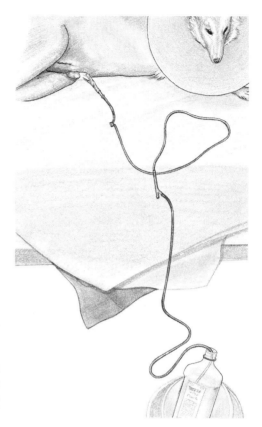

Figure 12-11 Collection apparatus in place for continuous urine drainage. Note collection container is below level of animal's urinary bladder.

Technical Action

5. Cleanse urethral orifice-catheter junction with soap and water twice daily and apply antimicrobial ointment to junction after cleansing.

Rationale/Amplification

5. Some drainage will occur at the exit point of the catheter. Catheter care helps prevent this exudate from entering the proximal urethra and bladder. The value of daily external urethral orifice care may be greater for high-risk patients. Care of the urethral orifice–catheter junction must include the application of antimicrobial ointment because cleansing with soap alone actually increased bacteriuria in some patients.

Technical Action	**Rationale/Amplification**
6. If urine flow stops, check position of animal and catheter. Try flushing catheter with 5 to 10 ml of sterile saline.	**6.** The animal may kink or compress the catheter when changing position. A flush of the catheter may be necessary to dislodge small clots or other debris in the catheter openings or lumen.
7. If continuous urine flow cannot be reestablished, replace catheter or reevaluate necessity for continuous urine drainage.	**7.** A free flow of urine is essential in preventing catheter-associated infection.

Bibliography

Biertuempfel PH, Ling GV, Ling GA: Urinary tract infection resulting from catheterization in healthy adult dogs. JAVMA 178 (9):989–991, 1981

Brunner LS, Suddarth DS: The Lippincott Manual of Nursing Practice, 3rd ed., Philadelphia, JB Lippincott, 1982

Burke JB, Jacobson JA, Garibaldi RA et al: Evaluation of daily meatal care with poly-antibiotic ointment in prevention of urinary catheter-associated bacteriuria. J Urol 129:331–334, Feb. 1983

Comer KM, Ling GV: Results of urinalysis and bacterial culture of canine urine obtained by antepubic cystocentesis, catheterization, and the midstream voided methods. JAVMA 179 (9):891–895, 1981

Crow SE: Hematuria: An algorithm for differential diagnosis. Compend Contin Educ Prac Vet II (12):941–948, 1980

Kirk RW, Bistner SI: Handbook of Veterinary Procedures and Emergency Treatment, 4th ed. Philadelphia, WB Saunders, 1985

Lees GE, Osborne CA: Urinary tract infections associated with the use and misuse of urinary catheters. Vet Clin North Am 9(4):713–727, 1979

Lees GE, Osborne CA, Stevens JB et al: Adverse effects caused by polypropylene and polyvinyl feline urinary catheters. Am J Vet Res 41(11):1836–1840, 1980

Lees GE, Osborne CA, Stevens JB, et al: Adverse effects of open indwelling urethral catheterization in clinically normal male cats. Am J Vet Res 42(5):825–833, 1981

Lees GE, Simpson RB, Green RA: Results of analyses and bacterial cultures of urine specimens obtained from clinically normal cats by three methods. JAVMA 184(4):449–454, 1984

Osborne CA, Klausner JS, Lees GE: Urinary tract infections: Normal and abnormal host defense mechanisms. Vet Clin North Am 9(4):587–609, 1979

Osborne CA, Klausner JS, Krawiec DR et al: Canine struvite urolithiasis: Problems and their dissolution. JAVMA 179(3):239–244, 1981

Osborne CA, Stevens JB: Handbook of Canine and Feline Urinalysis. St. Louis, MO, Ralston Purina, 1981

Osborne CA, Polzin DJ: Nonsurgical management of canine obstructive urolithopathy. Vet Clin North Am: Sm An Prac 16(2):333–349, 1986

Smith CW, Schiller AG, Smith AR, et al: Effects of indwelling urinary catheters in male cats. JAAHA 17:427–433, May/June, 1981

Stogdale L, Roos CJ: The use of the laryngoscope for bladder catheterization in the female dog. JAAHA 14:616–617, Sept/Oct 1978

Wolz GC: Urinary catheterization of the small animal patient, pp 207–215. Proceedings of 12th Annual Seminar for Veterinary Technicians, Western States Veterinary Conference, Las Vegas NV, Feb 21–23, 1983

Chapter 13

DIGITAL RECTAL EXAMINATION

If you don't know where you're going, you will probably end up somewhere else.

LAURENCE J. PETER

Digital rectal examination is the palpation of perineal and pelvic structures with one finger placed intrarectally through the anus.

Purpose

To identify diseases involving the rectum, anus, perineum, pelvic urethra, prostate, vagina, and pelvic bones

Specific Indications

1. Standard part of complete physical examination
2. Pelvic trauma
3. Stranguria
4. Hematuria
5. Pyuria
6. Tenesmus
7. Swellings or masses in perineal region
8. Hematochezia
9. Anal pruritus

Contraindications

1. Severe hematochezia
2. Painful tailbase

Equipment

- Examination gloves
- Lubricating jelly

Restraint and Positioning

Rectal palpation may be performed with the animal in a standing or recumbent position. The examiner should support the animal by gently cupping one hand under the animal's caudal abdomen, while the other gloved hand examines the rectal area. An assistant should restrain the animal by cradling the head and thorax in both arms.

Procedure

Technical Action

1. Place lubricant on index or middle finger of gloved hand.
2. Advance lubricated finger as far as possible into rectum (Fig. 13-1).

3. Systematically palpate pelvic canal and perineum proceeding from cranial to caudal. A recommended procedure is as follows:

Rationale/Amplification

1. The index finger should be used for small dogs and cats.
2. If there is a large amount of fecal material present, it should be removed before proceeding.
3. Proceeding from cranial to caudal in a uniform sequence helps to avoid errors of omission.

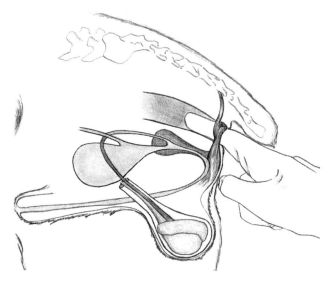

Figure 13-1 Placement of a gloved, lubricated finger in rectum for tactile inspection of the pelvic and perineal organs.

Technical Action

Slide finger lightly over the rectal mucosa for its entire circumference.

Palpate the following structures for location, size, consistency, and shape:

- Ventral aspect of sacrum
- Right ilium
- Right acetabulum
- Pubis
- Prostate or dorsal vaginal wall
- Left acetabulum
- Left ilium

Withdraw the finger ½ inch to 1½ inches and repeat circumferential palpation of

- Rectal mucosa
- Ventral aspect of coccygeal vertebrae
- Right perineal fascia
- Dorsal aspect of ischium
- Urethra
- Left perineal fascia

Continue caudally to the anus and palpate

- Anal sphincter muscles (note tone and reflex contraction)
- Anal sacs at 4 o'clock and 8 o'clock positions

The latter usually are best identified by squeezing them between the lubricated finger and the thumb, which is placed against the perineal skin.

4. Express contents of distended anal sacs (see also Chap. 14).

5. As finger is removed from the rectum, examine mucosa visually.

6. Examine soiled glove finger for blood, mucus, foreign materials, or parasites.

Rationale/Amplification

Particular attention should be paid to structures that protrude into or occlude the pelvic canal or the lumen of the rectum. In addition, note the animal's response when pressure is applied to each structure.

4. Collect secretions on cotton.

5. One cm to two cm of the rectal mucosa can be readily everted by gentle traction at the time of withdrawal.

6. This examination should consist of both inspection and palpation.

Chapter 14

ANAL SAC EXPRESSION AND CANNULATION

Kindness is the oil that takes the friction out of life.

M.A. HAMMARLUND

Anal sac expression is the manual removal of secretions that have accumulated in the animal's anal sacs. This procedure rarely is performed on cats. *Anal sac cannulation* is the insertion of a tube into the anal sac orifice.

Purposes

1. To remove malodorous secretions before bathing and grooming of dogs
2. To decrease irritation to the animal caused by distention or inflammation of its anal sacs
3. To instill medication in diseased anal sacs

Specific Indication

Anal pruritus

Complications

1. Rupture of abscessed anal sac
2. Perforation of rectum

Equipment Needed

- Cotton (or paper towels)
- Examination glove
- Lubricating jelly
- Skin disinfectant
- Prescribed medication

Restraint and Positioning

The dog should be restrained in the standing position by an assistant. A muzzle or Elizabethan collar may be needed. (see Chap. 1).

Procedure

Technical Action

1. Put on examination glove.

2. Express each anal sac externally by placing cotton over anus and pressing sac forward against perineum, while gently squeezing the sac with thumb and one or two fingers (Fig. 14-1).

Rationale/Amplification

1. Normal anal sac contents are malodorous. Use of an examination glove prevents soiling of the hands.

2. The anal sacs are located within the anal sphincter muscles on either side ventrolateral to the anus (4 o'clock and 8 o'clock positions). The duct of each sac opens just inside the anus.

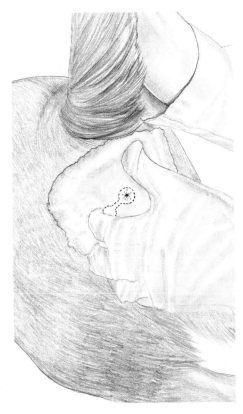

Figure 14-1 External expression of anal sac.

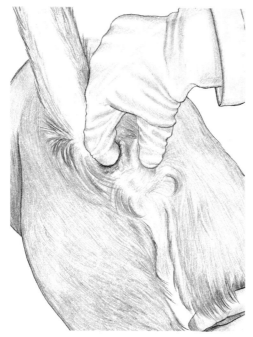

Figure 14-2 Internal expression of anal sac.

Technical Action

3. Express anal sacs more completely by inserting lubricated gloved index finger into rectum and gently milking contents of sac between finger and thumb dorsomedially into anal opening (Fig. 14-2).

4. Examine material expressed from anal sacs.
5. Invert glove and tie it in knot.

Rationale/Amplification

3. This is the preferred method of anal sac expression because it ensures emptying of the sacs. Rectal perforation, a very rare complication, can be prevented by gentle technique and adequate lubrication. If sacs cannot be expressed with light to moderate pressure, consider cannulation rather than applying more pressure.

4. Normal anal sacs contain a granular brown, malodorous material.
5. Enclosing anal sac material in this manner minimizes dispersion of odor in the examination room.

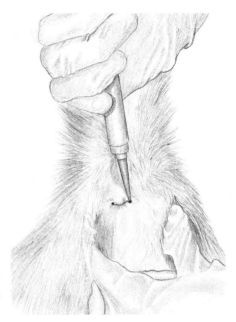

Figure 14-3 Flushing of anal sac by means of cannula inserted into anal sac duct.

Technical Action	**Rationale/Amplification**
6. If material expressed from anal sacs is purulent in appearance, identify duct openings and cannulate anal sac duct. Flush sacs several times with dilute povidone–iodine solution (Fig. 14-3).	6. Flushing with dilute povidone–iodine solution cleanses the interior aspect of the anal sacs. A 20-gauge polyethylene intravenous catheter is suitable in diameter and rigidity for cannulating anal sac ducts. Cannulation is facilitated by ejecting flushing solution through the cannula as it is introduced into the duct opening.
7. Instill prescribed medication into anal sacs.	7. Topical ointments, suitable for use in the ear, have been used to treat inflammation of the anal sac.
8. Note in patient's medical record any abnormalities observed or medication instilled.	8. Note date, time, medication, anal sac(s) affected, dosage, initials and comments.
9. Cleanse anus and surrounding skin with skin disinfectant.	9. Cleansing the area helps to dissipate odors lingering from the procedure.

Bibliography

Anal Sacs. Client education series. Indianapolis, Eli Lilly and Company

Muller GH, Kirk RW: Small Animal Dermatology. Philadelphia, WB Saunders, 1969

Pratt PW (ed): Medical Nursing for Animal Health Technicians. Santa Barbara, CA, American Veterinary Publications, 1985

Chapter 15

ENEMA

When a man has pity on all living creatures, then only is he noble.

BUDDHA

Enema is the infusion of fluid in the lower intestinal tract through the anus.

Purposes

1. To remove fecal material from the colon
2. To prepare for survey and contrast radiographic studies of abdomen and pelvis
3. To administer radiographic contrast media
4. To irrigate the colon in certain types of poisoning

Specific Indications

1. Constipation or obstipation
2. Some poisonings

Complications

1. Rupture of colon
2. Leakage of enema fluid into peritoneal cavity through already-ruptured gastrointestinal tract
3. Hemorrhage, in cases of ulcerative colitis

Equipment Needed

- Enema container with attached tubing and nozzle
- Enema solution (one or more of the following items)
  - Warm water
  - Glycerine and water (1 : 1)
  - Mild soap and water
  - Saline for irrigation
  - Commercial enema preparation

> NOTE: *Phosphate enema solutions should not be used in cats because these preparations may cause acute collapse associated with hypocalcemia in this species.*

- Examination glove
- Lubricating jelly

Restraint and Positioning

The animal is restrained in a standing position, usually in a wash basin or bathtub.

Procedure

Technical Action	Rationale/Amplification
1. Evaluate animal for evidence of abdominal pain or ulcerative colitis. If abdominal pain is present, eliminate the possibility of intestinal perforation or obstruction before proceeding.	1. Enemas are contraindicated in cases of intestinal obstruction or perforation because of the risk of forcing fecal material throughout the peritoneal cavity. Enemas may increase colonic bleeding in cases of ulcerative colitis.
2. Place prescribed warm enema solution in enema container.	2. Approximately 150 to 200 ml of an enema solution can be administered safely to an adult cat; a medium-sized or large dog can be given up to 1 liter. Warm solutions are preferred to cool solutions because the former are more readily retained and more comfortable for the animal.
3. Put on examination glove.	3. The glove will prevent soiling of the hand with feces.
4. Lubricate nozzle on end of enema tubing with lubricating jelly.	4. Lubrication of the nozzle facilitates atraumatic introduction of the tube into the rectum.

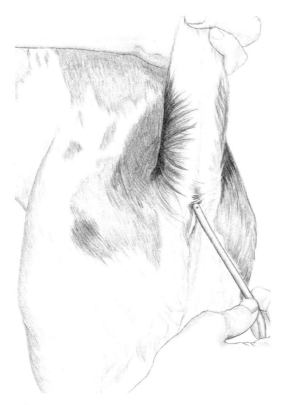

Figure 15-1 Inserting enema tube into animal's rectum.

Technical Action

5. Insert nozzle into animal's rectum (Fig. 15-1).

6. Place enema container higher than animal and permit solution to flow by gravity into animal's rectum.

7. After administering enema fluid, move animal immediately to suitable area for defecation.

8. Note in patient's medical record that enema was given.

Rationale/Amplification

5. The nozzle must be passed at least 2 inches cranial to the animal's anal sphincter.

6. Elevating the animal's hindquarters and gently gripping the sphincter around the nozzle will help to prevent enema fluid from escaping.

7. It may be necessary to administer two or three warm-water or saline enemas to cleanse the bowel adequately before a barium enema procedure.

8. Note date, time, type of enema, amount, initials, and comments.

Technical Action	**Rationale/Amplification**
9. For a barium enema: Anesthetize animal, position in right lateral recumbency, and place barium contrast material (20 to 30 ml/kg) into colon.	**9.** A cuffed rectal catheter is preferred to a routine enema nozzle for this procedure because anesthesia relaxes the anal sphincter and leakage of barium can occur readily. Contamination of the animal's hair or skin with contrast materials may result in radiographic artifacts that interfere with diagnosis.
10. Bathe animal's hindquarters or entire body.	**10.** The hair coat becomes soiled with feces during this procedure.

Bibliography

Brunner LS, Suddarth DS: The Lippincott Manual of Nursing Practice, 3rd ed. Philadelphia, JB Lippincott, 1982

Jones BV: Animal Nursing, Part 2. Oxford, Pergamon Press, 1966

Kirk RW, Bistner SI: Handbook of Veterinary Procedures and Emergency Treatment, 4th ed. Philadelphia, WB Saunders, 1985

Pratt PW (ed): Medical Nursing for Animal Health Technicians. Santa Barbara, CA, American Veterinary Publications, 1985

Part 2

SPECIALIZED CLINICAL PROCEDURES

The procedures described in this section are considered specialized because they require considerable preparation or have very specific indications. The reader should pay particular attention to those sections in applying these techniques.

As opposed to the "routine" procedures described in Part I, the specialized techniques frequently have significant inherent risk and may require specialized equipment. For the most part, however, the needed instruments are readily available and are not expensive.

Because these procedures are less commonly used in everyday practice, proficiency will take much longer than for routine techniques. Appropriate care and selection of these clinical tools will help the practicing veterinarian or technician to provide to clients and patients a more complete range and greater quality of diagnostic and therapeutic services.

When all else fails, read the instructions.

ANONYMOUS

Chapter 16

SKIN PREPARATION

We are held responsible not only for what we do, but for what we don't do.

CARL OSBORNE

Many of the procedures described in Part II are semi-invasive. Consequently, adequate disinfection of the skin is necessary to prevent sepsis. Methods of cleansing the skin of dogs and cats are described in almost every veterinary surgery text. For a thorough discussion of theory and principles of skin preparation, we refer our readers to those references.

Our preferred technique for skin preparation is described below. It is more than adequate for minimizing the probability of postoperative infection in all of the procedures included in this manual. Occasionally, some modifications are needed—such changes are described in the preparation section of each chapter for cases in which standard skin preparation technique is not appropriate.

Equipment Needed

- Animal hair clipper, with No. 10 or No. 40 blade
- 2" × 2" gauze sponges soaked in povidone–iodine surgical scrub
- 2" × 2" gauze sponges soaked in 70% alcohol
- Povidone–iodine solution
- Sponge forceps (optional)
- Surgical towels
- Fenestrated surgical drape
- Towel clamps (2 to 4)

Procedure

Technical Action	Rationale/Amplification
1. If the animal's skin is heavily soiled, consider bathing the whole animal before proceeding.	1. Bathing will help to minimize the chance of gross contamination of the operative site.
2. Immobilize the operative site.	2. Refer to recommended restraint measures for each procedure.
3. Clip hair close to skin from a large area around the operative site.	3. Do not skimp on area clipped. A wide margin is required to prevent contamination of the operative field. Clipped hairs should be less than 2-mm long.
4. Vacuum hair clippings and epithelial debris from entire area.	4. Do not touch the vacuum hose to the skin, as excessive suction may cause bruising.
5. Gently scrub the skin with sponges soaked in surgical scrub.	5. Start at the operative site and move the sponge outwardly toward the haired edges of the field, using a centrifugal spiral motion.
6. Remove the soap by wiping the operative site with alcohol-soaked gauze sponges.	6. Several sponges may be required.
7. Repeat Nos. 5 and 6 above at least two times.	7. The alternating soap and alcohol scrubs should be continued until no soil is visible on the used sponges.
8. After the last scrub, allow the operative field to air dry.	8. This delay allows the alcohol to kill more microorganisms.
9. Spray or paint the entire field with antiseptic solution.	9. Avoid applying excessive amounts of solution.
10. Place towels and drapes around operative site and secure to skin with towel clamps.	10. Towels and drapes help to prevent inadvertent contamination of instruments.

Bibliography

Catcott EJ (ed): Animal Health Technology. Santa Barbara, American Veterinary Publications, 1977

Knecht CD et al: Preparation of the operative site. In Knecht CD et al (ed): Fundamental Techniques in Veterinary Surgery, 2nd ed. Philadelphia, WB Saunders, 1981

Riser WH: Preparation of the patient's skin. In Archibald J (ed): Canine Surgery, 1st ed. Santa Barbara, American Veterinary Publications, 1965

Tracy DL, Warren RG: Small Animal Surgical Nursing. St Louis, CV Mosby, 1983

Chapter 17

INTUBATION

It's what you learn after you know it all that counts.

JOHN WOODEN

Intubation is the insertion of a tube into an organ or body cavity.

ENDOTRACHEAL INTUBATION

Endotracheal intubation is the placement of a tube that extends from the oral cavity into the trachea.

Purposes

1. To administer inhalation anesthetic drugs
2. To ensure a patent airway in unconscious animals
3. To administer oxygen
4. To provide ventilatory assistance

Complications

1. Trauma to teeth or mucous membranes of mouth, soft palate, pharynx, or larynx
2. Tracheal inflammation or necrosis
3. Subcutaneous emphysema secondary to tracheal trauma
4. Laryngospasm
5. Obstruction of the airway with secretions
6. Inadequate ventilation due to introduction of endotracheal tube into a bronchus
7. Aspiration of endotracheal tube

Equipment Needed

- Endotracheal tube of appropriate size and type (Table 17-1)
- Gauze strip, 12 to 20 inches long
- Sterile lubricating jelly
- 5-ml syringe
- Hemostat
- Laryngoscope or other light source
- Topical anesthetic spray (for cats)
- Additional equipment depending on circumstances
    Injectable anesthetic agents
    Inhalation anesthesia machine
    Ambu bag
    Emergency drugs

Restraint and Positioning

Endotracheal intubation is performed on dogs and cats who have been rendered unconscious by sedatives or anesthetic agents, trauma, or disease. Endotracheal intubation can be accomplished most easily when an assistant holds the animal in sternal recumbency. An animal also can be intubated while in lateral or dorsal recumbency. Large dogs may be intubated more easily while in lateral recumbency.

TABLE 17-1. Recommended Endotracheal Tube Sizes for Routine Use in Dogs and Cats*

Animal	Body Weight (lb)	Internal Diameter of Tube (mm)
Cat	2	3
	4	3.5–4
	8	4–4.5
Dog	5	5
	10	6
	15	6–7
	20	6–7
	25	6–8
	30	7–8
	35	7–8
	40	8–10
	45	8–10
	60	11–12

*Individual variations exist, and obesity must be taken into consideration. Some breeds (*e.g.,* Bulldogs) have relatively small tracheas for their body size, and some breeds (*e.g.,* Dachshunds) have large tracheas.

Procedure

Technical Action

1. Select endotracheal tube of appropriate diameter (see Table 17-1).

2. Premeasure length of tube against animal's neck (Fig. 17-1).

3. Check function of inflatable cuff, if present. Check that tube is clean and in good condition.

4. Lubricate tracheal end of tube with small amount of sterile lubricating jelly or water.
5. *Assistant:* (Fig. 17-2).
   a. Place animal in sternal recumbency.

Rationale/Amplification

1. Attempting to use a tube that is too large can cause trauma to the larynx or trachea. A tube that is too small will not provide an adequate airway.

2. Once in place the tip of the tube should be located midway between the larynx and the thoracic inlet. A longer tube is required for some surgical procedures (*e.g.,* cervical decompression).

3. Inflate the cuff with air, using a 5-ml syringe, and seal with stopper or hemostat. Observe and listen for leaks; submerge the cuff in water and observe for bubbles if in doubt about cuff seal.

4. Lubrication reduces irritation to the tracheal mucosa during intubation.

5. a. The assistant must hold the animal so that the head and neck are not twisted to either side.

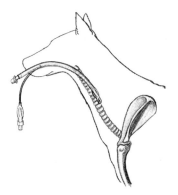

Figure 17-1 Premeasuring length of endotracheal tube required for animal.

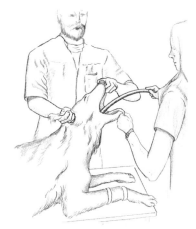

Figure 17-2 Restraint of animal for endotracheal intubation.

Technical Action

b. Extend animal's neck and open animal's mouth widely with one hand (or gauze strip) holding upper jaw.

c. Pull animal's tongue out of mouth with other hand.

6. *Operator:* Use laryngoscope to locate larynx (Fig. 17-3). If necessary, spray larynx of cat with topical anesthetic spray.

7. Depress epiglottis with tip of laryngoscope blade or endotracheal tube to examine arytenoid cartilages and vocal folds (Fig. 17-4).

8. Pass lubricated end of endotracheal tube through glottis and into trachea until tip of tube is midway between larynx and thoracic inlet. (Fig. 17-1) Check for correct placement of tube.

a. Auscult both sides of animal's chest for breath sounds.

b. Palpate neck for presence of two tubes.

Rationale/Amplification

b. Strips of gauze are particularly useful for holding the upper jaw of brachycephalic dogs.

c. Alternatively, the operator may grasp the tongue with one hand (see Fig. 17-2). A gauze sponge is useful for grasping a slippery tongue.

6. The use of a topical anesthetic is helpful in preventing laryngospasm during endotracheal intubation of the cat.

7. It is advisable to place the tip of a curved laryngoscope blade just anterior to the epiglottis in the cat so as to avoid laryngospasm, which can occur when the epiglottis is stimulated.

8. If the endotracheal tube is advanced too far, it can enter the right or left mainstem bronchus, thus eliminating ventilation of the other lung field. Palpation of two firm tubes in the neck indicates that the esophagus (rather than the trachea) has been intubated.

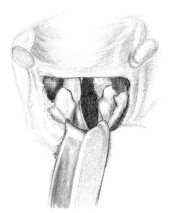

Figure 17-3 Laryngoscopic view of glottis.

Technical Action

   c. Directly palpate larynx and endotracheal tube if animal is well anesthetized.

9. Tie one single half-hitch knot around tube with gauze strip and then tie tube with quick release knot to upper jaw, lower jaw, or head behind ears (Fig. 17-5).

Rationale/Amplification

9. The tie should be placed posterior to the animal's canine teeth. The position of the gauze tie will depend on whether a procedure is to be performed in the head or neck region.

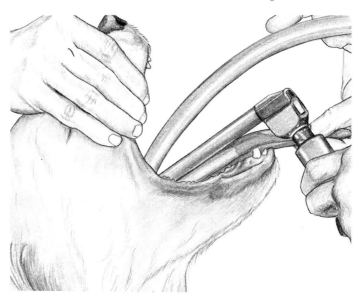

Figure 17-4 Use of laryngoscope to inspect glottis.

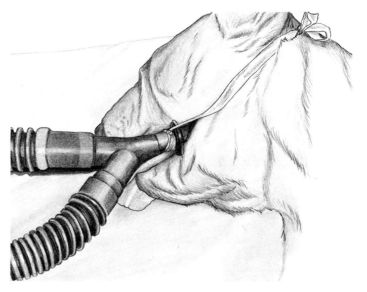

Figure 17-5 Endotracheal tube tied in place.

Technical Action

10. Connect endotracheal tube to inhalation anesthetic machine, Ambu bag, or respirator when required.

11. Inflate cuff of endotracheal tube with sufficient air to seal area between tube and trachea (Fig. 17-7).

Rationale/Amplification

10. The Ambu bag is used for manual ventilation of an animal in respiratory arrest (Fig. 17-6).

11. Overinflation of the cuff can cause tracheal inflammation and necrosis. If more than 5 ml of air is needed to inflate the cuff in a dog (or 2 ml in a cat), replace endotracheal tube with one of larger diameter. A leak should be heard around the tube when one is manually ventilating an animal with more than twice its tidal volume. This leak will act as a "safety valve" and protect the lungs from overinflation.

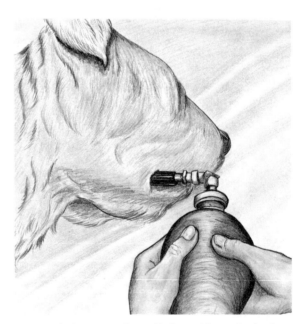

Figure 17-6 Manual ventilation with an Ambu bag.

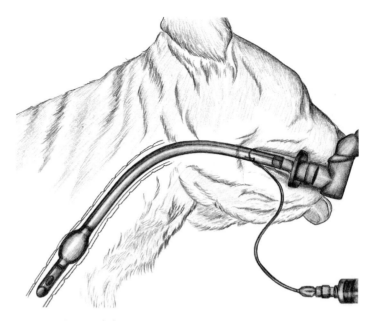

Figure 17-7 Inflating cuff of endotracheal tube.

Technical Action

12. While animal is intubated, observe frequently for:
    a. kinking of endotracheal tube due to malpositioning of neck,
    b. obstruction of endotracheal tube with secretions, and
    c. biting of endotracheal tube (because of return of reflexes).

13. Loosen tie on tube as reflexes begin to return. Deflate cuff and remove tube (extubate) when swallowing reflex has returned.

14. Position animal with head, neck, and tongue extended and continue to observe until animal is fully conscious.

Rationale/Amplification

12. Indications of adequate ventilation include normal pink color of mucous membranes and clear lung sounds on auscultation. It is sometimes necessary to remove secretions by tracheal suctioning through the endotracheal tube. An animal must be observed closely while regaining consciousness so that it does not bite through the endotracheal tube and aspirate it.

13. Removing an endotracheal tube with an inflated cuff is traumatic to the trachea and larynx and should be avoided.

14. In the semiconscious state following anesthesia, an animal can die as a result of airway obstruction.

CHEST TUBE PLACEMENT

Chest tube placement is the insertion of a flexible catheter into the pleural cavity.

Purposes

1. To remove fluids or air continuously or repeatedly from the chest
2. To infuse certain medications into the chest

Specific Indications

1. Pneumothorax
2. Pleural effusion

Complications

1. Leakage of room air into chest tube with resulting pneumothorax
2. Pleural inflammation or infection
3. Puncture of intercostal artery
4. Laceration of lung with resulting hemothorax or pneumothorax
5. Laceration of heart or great vessels

Equipment Needed

- Sterile chest tube: rubber or soft vinyl urethral catheter or commercial chest tube, 14 F or larger
- Cotton
- Clipper with No. 40 blade
- Skin preparation materials
    Povidone–iodine surgical scrub
    Povidone–iodine solution
    Sterile gauze sponges (2″ × 2″)
- Drugs and equipment for general anesthesia, or 2% lidocaine for local anesthesia in critically ill animals
- Cap and mask
- Sterile surgical equipment
    Drapes
    Gown
    Surgeon's gloves
    Gauze sponges
    Scalpel blade and handle
    Scissors
    Two curved hemostats
    Suture material: monofilament, nonabsorbable
    3-way stopcock and catheter adapter
    Straight hemostat
    50-ml syringe

• Bandaging material
    Sterile gauze sponges
    Antimicrobial ointment
    Gauze bandage
    Adhesive tape (2-inch wide) or elastic adhesive bandage

Restraint and Positioning

General anesthesia is preferred for the maintenance of strict asepsis during chest tube placement. If the animal's critical condition precludes general anesthesia, the area for chest tube placement, including the pleura, is infiltrated with 2% lidocaine. The animal should be positioned in lateral recumbency.

Procedure

Technical Action

1. Clip and surgically prepare skin over lateral thorax from fifth to ninth intercostal spaces using povidone–iodine surgical scrub and solution.
2. If general anesthesia cannot be used, infiltrate skin, subcutaneous tissue, intercostal muscles, and pleura with 2% lidocaine.
3. Don cap, mask, sterile gown, and gloves. Place sterile drapes around chest tube insertion site.
4. Cut additional holes in chest tube, if necessary. Seal end of chest tube with catheter adapter and 3-way stopcock.

5. Make small incision in skin at level of midthorax over eighth or ninth intercostal space.

6. Using curved hemostat, tunnel cranially through subcutaneous tissue to sixth or seventh intercostal space (Fig. 17-8).

Rationale/Amplification

1. Failure to cleanse the skin thoroughly before chest tube insertion can result in infection.

2. A total of 2 to 5 ml of lidocaine may be needed to provide adequate local anesthesia.

3. Strict attention to asepsis is recommended.

4. It is advantageous to have several holes in the tube to decrease the chance of blockage of the tube with secretions. The chest tube should be sealed during insertion to prevent room air from entering the chest.

5. The skin incision should be two intercostal spaces caudal to the intended insertion site of the chest tube.

6. The subcutaneous tunnel is made with the hemostat by gentle blunt dissection. The tunnel must be wide enough to accommodate a second hemostat and a chest tube.

Technical Action

7. Force closed hemostat into thoracic cavity, keeping close to cranial edge of seventh or eighth rib (Fig. 17-9).

8. Spread jaws of hemostat and leave in place.

Rationale/Amplification

7. The intercostal arteries are located along the caudal edge of each rib and must be avoided to minimize the chance of severe hemorrhage.

8. Spreading the jaws of the hemostat prevents the pleura and intercostal muscles from occluding the puncture site.

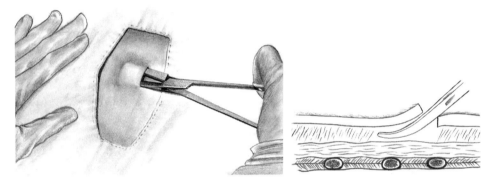

Figure 17-8   Formation of subcutaneous tunnel for chest tube.

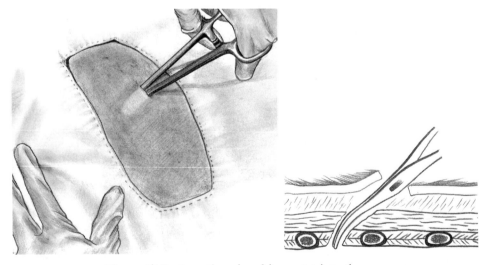

Figure 17-9   Inserting closed hemostat into thorax.

Technical Action

9. Place tip of chest tube between jaws of second curved hemostat. Advance second hemostat through subcutaneous tunnel so that tube tip just enters thoracic cavity (Fig. 17-10).

10. Open jaws of second hemostat and manually advance chest tube well into thoracic cavity.

11. Remove both hemostats.

Rationale/Amplification

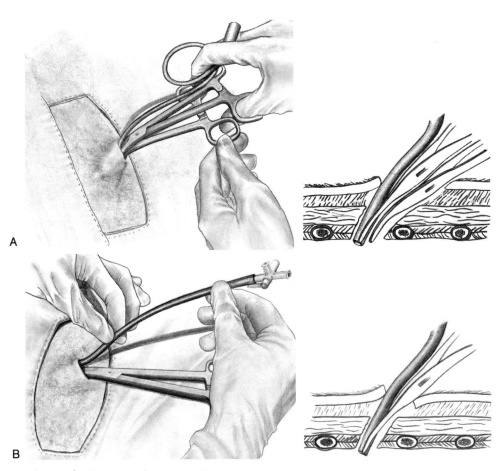

Figure 17-10 (*A*) and (*B*) Inserting chest tube into thoracic opening made with closed hemostat.

Technical Action

12. Hold sponge over subcutaneous tunnel while aspirating chest tube with 50-ml syringe (Fig. 17–11).

13. Place purse-string suture through skin edges around exit point of chest tube from skin (Fig. 17-12 *A*).

14. Make adhesive tape "butterfly" around chest tube and suture "butterfly" to skin with simple interrupted sutures (Fig. 17-12 *B*).

15. Place antimicrobial ointment and sterile gauze sponge over skin incision.

16. Bandage chest tube in place by completely encircling thorax with gauze and adhesive tape or elastic adhesive bandage.

17. Place straight hemostat on chest tube proximal to stopcock, and incorporate jaws of hemostat into bandage (Fig. 17-13).

Rationale/Amplification

12. If no fluid or air can be aspirated, the tube should be advanced or withdrawn slightly until patency is ensured.

14. The adhesive tape helps to anchor the chest tube in position.

16. The bandage must permit the animal to breathe easily, but it should be secure.

17. The hemostat is additional protection against iatrogenic pneumothorax should the stopcock become dislodged.

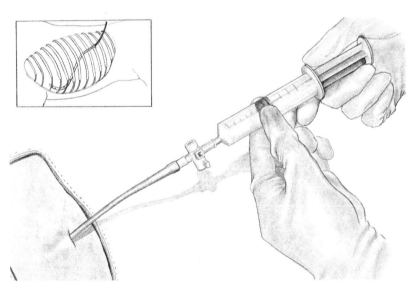

Figure 17-11 Aspirating chest tube to ensure correct placement.

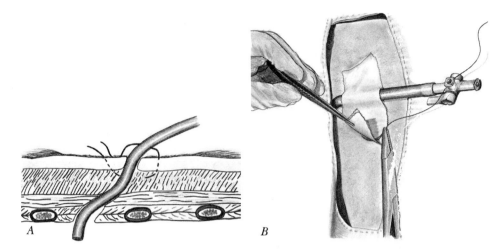

Figure 17-12 (*A*) Purse-string suture around exit point of chest tube. (*B*) Adhesive tape "butterfly" around chest tube sutured to skin.

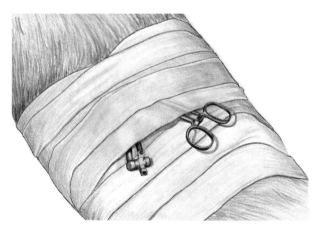

Figure 17-13 Bandage covering chest tube and jaws of hemostat.

Technical Action	**Rationale/Amplification**
18. Aspirate chest tube at prescribed intervals, moving animal into various positions if necessary.	18. It is inadvisable to leave an animal with a chest tube in place unattended. Note date, time, volume and appearance of material aspirated, initials, and comments in animal's medical record.

OROGASTRIC INTUBATION

Orogastric intubation is the placement of a tube that extends from the oral cavity into the stomach.

Purposes

1. To administer medication and certain radiographic contrast materials
2. To remove stomach contents
3. To perform gastric lavage (see Chap. 18, pp. 169–171)
4. To administer nutrients (*e.g.,* to puppies and kittens)

Complications

1. Administration of materials into respiratory tract owing to incorrect placement of tube
2. Esophageal trauma
3. Gastric irritation
4. Gastric perforation

Equipment Needed

- Stomach tube
    12 F rubber urethral catheter for kittens and puppies
    18 F rubber urethral catheter for adult cats and dogs up to 40 lb
    Foal stomach tube for dogs > 40 lb
- speculum
    Commercial canine mouth speculum or roll of 2-inch wide adhesive tape
    1-inch wide wooden dowel with center hole for cats
- Adhesive tape or ballpoint pen for marking stomach tube
- Lubricating jelly
- Syringe containing 5 ml of sterile saline
- Syringe or funnel for material to be administered

Restraint and Positioning

Restrain the animal in sternal recumbency.

Procedure

Technical Action	Rationale/Amplification
1. Premeasure stomach tube by holding it next to animal. When tip is at level of last rib, mark point on tube at oral opening with ballpoint pen or adhesive tape (Fig. 17-14).	1. When premeasuring the tube, one must follow the curvature of the neck in order to accurately estimate the length of the esophagus.

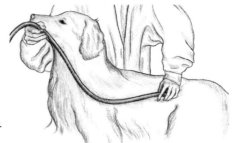

Figure 17-14 Premeasuring length of stomach tube required for animal.

Technical Action

2. Moisten tip of stomach tube with lubricating jelly.

3. Insert speculum into animal's mouth and hold animal's jaws closed on speculum.

4. Pass lubricated stomach tube through speculum and advance to premarked point (Fig. 17-15). If possible, advance tip of tube past larynx while animal is exhaling.

Rationale/Amplification

2. Lubrication of the tube helps to minimize the possibility of esophageal trauma while the tube is passed.

3. Some cats object so strenuously to this procedure that it cannot be performed without anesthesia. Nasogastric intubation should be considered for such cats.

4. Inability to pass the tube to the premeasured length may indicate that:

   a. it has been inserted into the trachea,

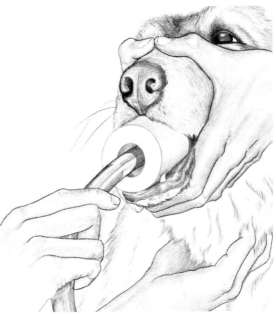

Figure 17-15 Inserting lubricated stomach tube through tape speculum.

Technical Action	Rationale/Amplification
	b. there is obstruction of the esophagus, or
	c. gastric volvulus has occurred, preventing entry of the tube into the stomach.
5. Check proper placement of stomach tube as follows: a. palpate tube within neck, b. smell end of tube for gastric odors, c. blow into tube while assistant auscults stomach for gurgling, d. administer 5 ml of sterile saline by the stomach tube and observe for cough.	5. If the tube is in the esophagus, two tubes (the stomach tube and the trachea) should be palpable in the neck. If there is any evidence that the tube has been inserted into the trachea, remove the tube and reinsert it.
6. Administer materials prescribed or remove gastric contents. Then administer 3 to 8 ml of water to flush tube.	6. If orogastric intubation is performed on an unconscious animal, a cuffed endotracheal tube should be inserted before passing the stomach tube. This will prevent aspiration of any material regurgitated around the tube.
7. Before removing tube, seal end of tube with thumb.	7. This will help to prevent leakage of any material remaining in the tube into the pharynx when the tube is removed.
8. Note in animal's medical record that procedure was performed.	8. Note date, time, procedure, any materials removed or administered, initials, and comments.

NASOGASTRIC INTUBATION OF THE CAT

Nasogastric intubation is the placement of a tube that extends through an external naris, the nasal cavity, pharynx and esophagus, and into the stomach. This procedure is of practical use mainly in the adult cat because of the relatively short nasal passage in that species. The procedure cannot be performed on kittens or on any cat with an obstruction of the nasal cavity.

Purposes

1. To administer medication and radiographic contrast materials
2. To administer nutritional supplements and water

Complications

1. Administration of materials into the respiratory tract
2. Esophageal trauma
3. Gastric irritation

Equipment Needed

- Nasogastric tube: infant feeding tube or 21-gauge butterfly catheter (winged infusion set) with needle assembly cut-off
- Topical ophthalmic anesthetic
- Lubricating jelly
- Syringe with 1 ml of sterile saline
- Syringe for material to be administered
- Bandaging material if catheter is to remain in place
    Gauze, 2 inches wide
    Adhesive tape or elastic adhesive bandage, 2 inches wide
    Injection cap

Restraint and Positioning

The cat is held in a sitting position or in sternal recumbency by an assistant.

Procedure

Technical Action

1. Instill four or five drops of topical ophthalmic anesthetic into one nostril (Fig. 17-16).

Rationale/Amplification

1. The cat may sneeze at first.

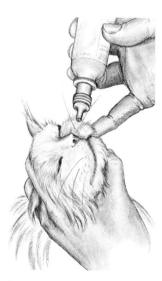

Figure 17-16 Instilling topical ophthalmic anesthetic into cat's nostril.

Technical Action

2. Wait 2 to 3 minutes, then instill two or three more drops of topical ophthalmic anesthestic into same nostril.

3. Apply a small amount of lubricating jelly to tip of nasogastric tube.

4. Hold cat's head with one hand and use other hand to insert tube into ventromedial aspect of anesthetized nostril (Fig. 17-17).

5. Advance tube approximately 20 to 25 cm.

6. Check proper placement of nasogastric tube by instilling 1 ml of sterile saline into tube.

7. Administer prescribed materials and flush nasogastric tube with 1 or 2 ml of water.

8. Bandage catheter in place to side of cat's neck if repeated nasogastric intubation is anticipated and cat will tolerate leaving tube in place (Fig. 17-18).

Rationale/Amplification

2. During instillation of the topical ophthalmic anesthetic into the nostril, the cat's head should be positioned with its nose toward the ceiling.

3. Lubrication of the tube helps to minimize irritation to the nasal cavity, esophagus, and stomach during passage of the tube.

4. The cat can feel the pressure of the tube and may resist the procedure slightly.

5. If the tube is difficult to pass, try rotating it gently before advancing it farther.

6. If the cat coughs, it should be assumed that the tube is in the trachea and the tube should be removed and reinserted. Vigorous laryngeal reflexes in cats usually prevent inadvertent intubation of the trachea.

8. Severely debilitated cats usually will tolerate long-term placement of the tube. The end of the catheter should be covered to prevent aspiration of air into the cat's stomach.

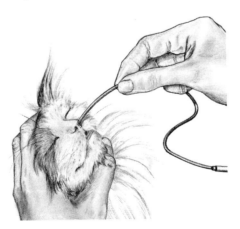

Figure 17-17 Inserting nasogastric tube into cat's naris.

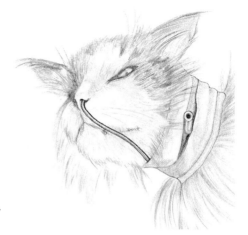

Figure 17-18 Nasogastric tube bandaged in place.

Technical Action

9. Before removing tube, seal end of tube with thumb or finger.

10. Note in animal's medical record that procedure was performed.

Rationale/Amplification

9. This will help to prevent leakage of any material remaining in the tube into the pharynx when the tube is removed.

10. Note date, time, procedure, any materials administered, initials, and comments.

PHARYNGOSTOMY TUBE PLACEMENT

A *pharyngostomy tube* is placed such that it extends from the lateral wall of the oropharynx into the esophagus or stomach.

Purpose

To administer nutrients and medications orally over days or weeks to an animal that is unable to eat because of debilitation, oral lesions, or head trauma, but whose gastrointestinal tract is functioning normally

Complications

1. Vomiting or regurgitation
2. Aspiration pneumonia
3. Pharyngitis, laryngitis
4. Esophagitis or esophageal perforation
5. Distension of stomach with air
6. Gastritis

Equipment Needed

- Sterile pharyngostomy tube: soft rubber or vinyl feeding tube
  18 F for cat or small dog
  Larger sizes for dogs > 35 lb
- Commerical mouth speculum for dog or cat
- Cotton
- Clipper with No. 40 blade
- Anesthetic drugs and equipment for general anesthesia
- Skin preparation materials
  Povidone–iodine surgical scrub
  Povidone–iodine solution
  Sterile gauze sponges (2″ × 2″)
- Sterile surgical equipment
  Surgeon's gloves
  Scalpel blade and handle
  2 Kelly or Crile curved hemostats
  Suture material: monofilament, nonabsorbable
  Scissors
  Gauze sponges
- Bandaging material
  Sterile gauze sponges
  Antimicrobial ointment
  Gauze bandage
  Adhesive tape, 1 inch wide
  Adhesive tape or elastic adhesive bandage, 2 inches wide
  Stopper for pharyngostomy tube

Restraint and Positioning

General anesthesia is needed for placement of a pharyngostomy tube. The animal is positioned in lateral recumbency.

Procedure

Technical Action	Rationale/Amplification
1. Clip and surgically prepare skin over lateral pharyngeal wall with povidone–iodine surgical scrub and solution.	
2. Place speculum in animal's mouth.	
3. Premeasure pharyngostomy tube by holding it next to animal (Fig. 17-19).	3. Use either the eighth or the thirteenth rib as the point for placement of the tip of the tube.

Technical Action   **Rationale/Amplification**

NOTE: *Some controversy exists over whether a pharyngostomy tube should terminate in the midesophagus or the stomach. Some authors advise against the use of these tubes altogether. We believe they can be effective when used judiciously.*

4. Carefully palpate hyoid apparatus with finger in mouth and other hand on external part of neck (Fig. 17-20).

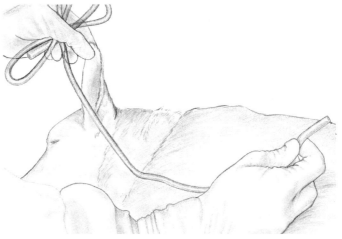

Figure 17-19 Premeasuring pharyngostomy tube.

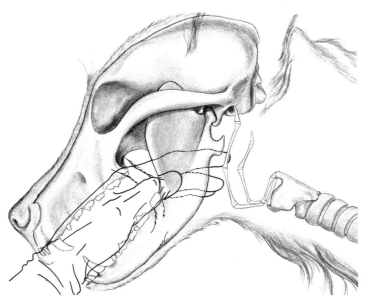

Figure 17-20 Palpating hyoid apparatus.

Technical Action

5. Insert hemostat into mouth and push jaws laterally against pharyngeal wall immediately cranial to hyoid apparatus.

6. Make small incision through skin on lateral aspect of neck immediately cranial to hyoid apparatus where hemostat jaws protrude (Fig. 17-21).

7. Gently force hemostat through lateral pharyngeal wall and skin incision (Fig. 17-22).

8. Grasp closed end of pharyngostomy tube in hemostat jaws and pull it through incision into pharynx (Fig. 17-23).

9. Push pharyngostomy tube down esophagus to predetermined point with fingers.

Rationale/Amplification

5. By keeping one or two fingers of one hand in animal's mouth, one can guide the hemostat into proper position within the pharynx.

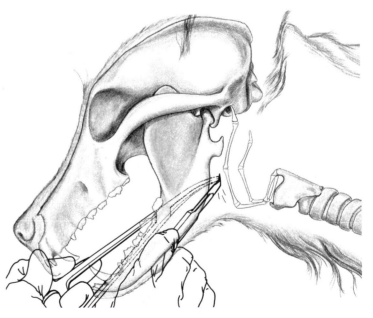

Figure 17-21 Incising skin over hemostat jaws.

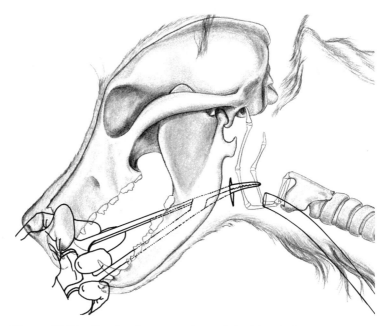

Figure 17-22   Forcing hemostat through incision in lateral pharynx.

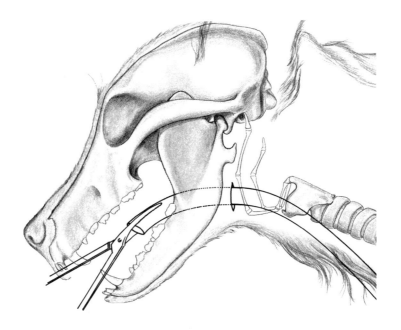

Figure 17-23   Pulling pharyngostomy tube into pharynx with hemostat.

Technical Action

10. Check that pharyngostomy tube lies lateral and dorsal to larynx.

11. Make adhesive tape "butterfly" around pharyngostomy tube and suture butterfly to skin with simple interrupted sutures (Fig. 17-24).

12. Place antimicrobial ointment and sterile gauze sponge over skin incision.

13. Bandage pharyngostomy tube in place by encircling neck completely with gauze and adhesive tape or elastic adhesive bandage, leaving 1 or 2 inches of stoppered tube protruding from bandage (Fig. 17-25).

14. X-ray animal to ensure correct position of pharyngostomy tube.

Rationale/Amplification

10. Proper positioning of the pharyngostomy tube within the pharynx should prevent its acting as an obstruction or irritation to the larynx.

11. Adhesive tape helps to anchor the pharyngostomy tube in position.

13. An Elizabethan collar should be placed on the animal if the animal frequently attempts to scratch at the bandage.

14. Some potential malpositioning problems include advancing the tube too far, knotting it within stomach, or doubling the tube back on itself.

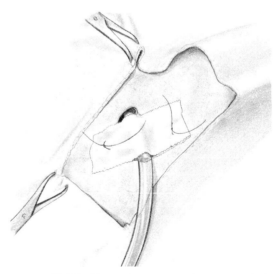

Figure 17-24 Pharyngostomy tube secured in place by adhesive tape butterfly sutured to skin.

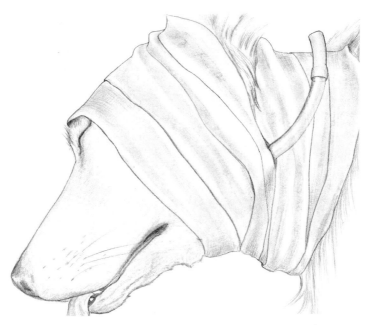

Figure 17-25 Bandage covering pharyngostomy tube.

Technical Action

15. When animal is fully awake, test animal's tolerance of feeding by pharyngostomy tube by administering small amounts of water every hour.

16. If animal does not regurgitate or vomit, proceed with nutritional program at prescribed intervals.

Rationale/Amplification

15. Some animals may vomit or regurgitate initially. If this problem persists, the pharyngostomy tube should be removed and an alternative method of alimentation instituted.

16. The tube should be flushed with 2 to 6 ml of water before and after each use and stoppered between feedings.

Bibliography

Bohning RH: Pharyngostomy for oral maintenance. In Bojrab MJ (ed): Current Techniques in Small Animal Surgery, pp 101–103. Philadelphia, Lea & Febiger, 1975

Dodman NH, Seeler DC, Court MH: Aging changes in the geriatric dog and their impact on anesthesia. Comp Contin Educ for Prac Vet 6(12):1106–1112, 1984

Ford RB: Nasogastric intubation in the cat. Comp Contin Educ for AHT 1(1):29–33, 1980

Harvey CE, O'Brien, JA: Management of respiratory emergencies in small animals. Vet Clin North Am 2(2):243–258, 1972

Kirk RW, Bistner SI: Handbook of Veterinary Procedures and Emergency Treatment, 4th ed. Philadelphia, WB Saunders, 1985

Lantz GC, Cantwell HD, VanVleet JF et al: Pharyngostomy tube induced esophagitis in the dog: An experimental study. JAAHA 19(2):207–212, 1983

Sawyer DC, Evans AT, DeYoung DJ et al: Anesthetic Principles and Techniques. East Lansing, Michigan State University Press, 1981

Walshaw R: Personal communication, 1983

Warren RG: Small Animal Anesthesia. St. Louis, CV Mosby, 1983

Chapter 18

GASTRIC LAVAGE

If you don't learn from your mistakes, there's no sense making them.

HERBERT V. PROCHNOW

✳ *Gastric lavage* is the flushing and evacuation of stomach contents.

Specific Indications

1. Ingestion of poisonous substances
2. Inadvertent overdosage of medication
3. Gastric dilatation

Complications

1. Aspiration of gastric contents into respiratory tract
2. Inadvertent instillation of fluid into respiratory tract
3. Trauma to the pharynx or larynx

Equipment Needed

- Orogastric tube
- Plastic tubing adapter
- Isotonic diluting fluids
- Vacuum/suction system (if possible)

Restraint and Positioning

The degree of restraint required depends on the status of the patient. An agitated patient (*e.g.,* strychnine poisoning victim) may require general anesthesia, whereas a comatose animal requires no further restraint. An animal with the ideal level of restraint is tranquil, immobile, but conscious.

The animal is <u>held in sternal recumbency or in a sitting position while the</u> <u>tube is passed and fluid is instilled.</u> After the stomach is filled, the head is held upright while the torso is rolled so that it assumes <u>left lateral recumbency.</u> The <u>procedure requires two persons.</u>

Procedure

Technical Action	Rationale/Amplification
1. <u>Obtain a detailed history and examine the label of any suspected toxin, if possible.</u> *V. important!*	**1.** Several types of poisons or compounds should not be treated by gastric lavage. Their labels generally will indicate same. If in doubt, <u>consult National Animal Poison Control Center (217-333-3611).</u> *There is also a hotline (1-800 #)*

✳ NOTE: *Speed is of great importance. In most instances, gastric lavage is only valu-* <u>*able when performed within 1 hour of toxin ingestion.*</u>

2. Perform a rapid but thorough physical examination.	**2.** Particular attention to pupillary size and response, swallowing reflexes, and alertness may help in deciding what additional supportive care is needed.
3. If animal is unconscious, insert endotracheal tube and inflate cuff.	**3.** Endotracheal intubation prevents inadvertent aspiration of fluid. See Chapter 17, pp. 143–149.
4. <u>Pass an orogastric tube. Be sure of its proper position before proceeding.</u> *Down the esophagus, not the trachea.*	**4.** See Chapter 17, pp. 156–158.
5. <u>Evacuate all stomach contents.</u>	**5.** If a suction line is available, attach to orogastric tube via plastic adapter. If a vacuum line is *not* available, establish the siphon effect by holding the end of the tubing below body level and applying suction by bulb or by mouth. (Be careful not to ingest any stomach contents!)
6. Save an <u>aliquot</u> of the first collection for possible analysis.	
7. <u>Attach funnel or infusion set.</u>	
8. <u>Rapidly infuse approximately 5 to 6 ml of an isotonic electrolyte solution per kg of body weight.</u>	**8.** This volume should fill the stomach to approximately two thirds of its maximum volume.

Technical Action

9. Holding the animal's head high, roll the torso into left lateral recumbency.

10. Gently rock the animal back and forth several times by raising the feet several inches off the table or floor.

11. Evacuate stomach contents as in No. 5.

12. Repeat Nos. 7 through 11 several times.

13. Infuse antidote or absorbent through tube, if indicated. *CHARCOAL INFUSION (LAST STEP)*

14. Place thumb over end of tube and withdraw tube slowly by applying gentle, steady traction.

Rationale/Amplification

9. This procedure allows bathing of the fundic portion of the stomach while preventing aspiration of fluids.

10. Rocking may help to dislodge viscous fluids or solid materials adhering to the gastric mucosa.

12. If the animal becomes unruly or uncomfortable, discontinue flushing temporarily. Recommence within a few minutes, if possible.

14. Observe for swallowing reflex. If no swallowing is seen, observe the animal closely for vomiting or regurgitation. Consider placing an inflated endotracheal tube.

Bibliography

Kirk RW, Bistner SI: Handbook of Veterinary Procedures and Emergency Treatment, 3rd ed. Philadelphia, WB Saunders, 1981

Walshaw R: Personal communication, 1983

RD. for wed.

Chapter 19

DENTAL PROPHYLAXIS

The gem cannot be polished without friction, nor man perfected without trials.

CONFUCIUS

Dental prophylaxis is a series of procedures by which calculus and stain are removed from the crowns of the teeth and the enamel surfaces are polished.

Purposes

1. To remove calculus and stain from teeth
2. To improve condition of gingival tissues
3. To control periodontal disease
4. To treat halitosis caused by calculus and debris adhering to dental surfaces

Complications

1. Injury to gingival tissues
2. Damage to enamel
3. Bacteremia

Equipment Needed

 Endotracheal tube
• Apparatus and agents for general anesthesia
• Gauze sponges (2″ × 2″)
• Dental instruments (Fig. 19-1)
  Curette
  Universal scaler
  Prophy angle
• Ultrasonic scaler (optional)

- Polishing equipment
    Dental engine with prophy attachment for power-driven dental drill or commercial polishing apparatus
    Prophy cups
    Dental pumice paste (medium and fine)
- Plastic rinse bottle containing water

Restraint and Positioning

Successful dental prophylaxis requires that the animal be under general anesthesia. A routine presurgical evaluation should precede the administration of the anesthetic. The anesthetized animal is positioned in lateral recumbency with its head tilted slightly downward.

Procedure

Technical Action

1. If prophylactic antibiotics are prescribed, give first dose 1 to 4 hours before procedure depending on route of medication administration (oral versus parenteral).

Rationale/Amplification

1. A transient bacteremia may occur after any dental procedure.

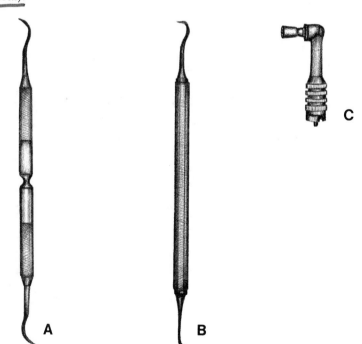

Figure 19-1   Dental instruments: (*A*) curette, (*B*) universal scaler, and (*C*) prophy angle.

prophy cup
(rubber)

Technical Action

2. Anesthetize animal and place endotracheal tube. Check endotracheal tube for evidence of leaks around tube or cuff.

3. Carefully examine gingival tissues and all surfaces of teeth.

4. Evaluate occlusion.

5. Check for swelling and hyperemia of gingival edge, presence of fistulas, fractured teeth, retained deciduous teeth, deformed teeth, and asymmetry in calculus.

6. Place animal's head over grid or towels, and tilt head so that rostral end of muzzle is slightly lower than the rest of the head.

7. Wear mask and goggles, especially if ultrasonic scaler is to be used.

use paper towels

8. Remove accumulations of calculus from crowns of teeth.

 a. If ultrasonic scaler is used, ensure adequate water spray by adjusting water flow such that one drop of water per second drips from "resting" instrument. Keep tip of instrument in motion along dental surfaces (Fig. 19-2).

Rationale/Amplification

2. Use of an endotracheal tube with a properly inflated cuff will help to decrease the possibility of aspiration of water or debris during the procedure.

4. When mouth is closed, the lower canine tooth should fit caudal to the upper lateral incisor and mesial to the upper canine tooth.

5. Retained deciduous teeth and most deformed teeth should be extracted. A root canal procedure or extraction is required for abscessed teeth or fractured teeth with exposed pulp. Asymmetrical calculus accumulation may indicate reluctance of the animal to chew on the side with the heavier deposits.

6. The slight downward tilt of the animal's head helps reduce the risk of aspiration of water used for rinsing during the procedure.

7. The aerosol created by the ultrasonic scaler is likely to contain bacteria that could be pathogenic for human beings.

8. Calculus may be removed by use of an ultrasonic scaler or hand-held scaling instruments.

 a. Heat is generated by the high frequency vibrations of the instrument along the tooth. The water spray prevents thermal damage to the tooth and helps to remove dislodged calculus. Minimize the possibility of etching the enamel or damaging the tooth by excessive heat by never leaving the instrument on a tooth for more than 10 to 15 seconds at a time.

Technical Action	**Rationale/Amplification**
b. If hand-held scaling instrument is used, hold instrument like a pencil and pull calculus from tooth with powerful short dislodging strokes (Fig. 19-3).	b. Hand-held scaling instruments are essential for removing calculus between teeth. Heavy accumulations of calculus may be cracked before scaling with a tartar forceps.

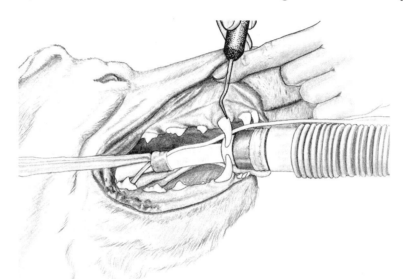

Figure 19-2 Use of ultrasonic scaler on crown of tooth.

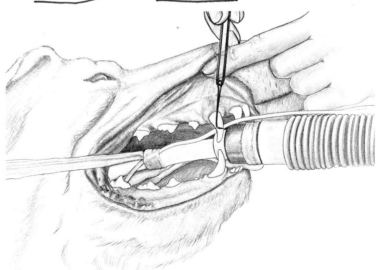

Figure 19-3 Use of hand-held scaler.

Technical Action

9. Using short upward dislodging movements, scrape away subgingival calculus on roots of teeth with a dental curette.

10. Insert dental curette into crevice between tooth and gingiva with cutting edge toward gingival wall. Remove debris and diseased tissue by upward strokes of curette (Fig. 19-4).

11. Polish crown of each tooth using polishing device at low speed, taking care to avoid gingival edge. Use quick, light touch to polish tooth with dental pumice paste. Move instrument from tooth to tooth every few seconds (Fig. 19-5).

Rationale/Amplification

9. The ultrasonic scaler should not be used under the gumline because it can easily damage the periodontal ligaments that anchor the tooth in the bone.

10. The purpose of gingival curettage is to remove dead epithelium and debris, thus stimulating healing of the inflamed gingival tissue. Double-edged dental curettes are available, permitting stimultaneous gingival curettage and removal of calculus from the tooth root.

11. Polishing removes stains and plaque and smooths the tooth surface, thus slowing subsequent accumulation of plaque. Abrasion of enamel during polishing can be prevented by keeping the instrument on a single tooth for only a few seconds and by avoid-

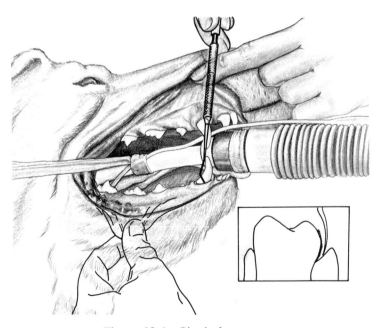

Figure 19-4 Gingival curettage.

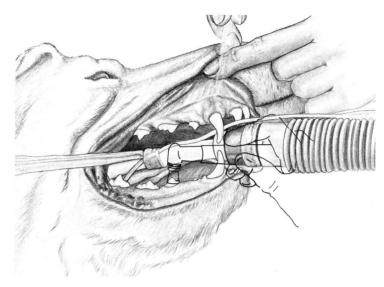

Figure 19-5 Polishing crown of tooth.

Technical Action

Rationale/Amplification

ing excessive pressure or application of too much pumice at
any one point.

12. Rinse pumice, blood, and debris
from teeth by using a gentle
stream of water.

13. Instruct client in regular care of
animal's teeth.

✱13. The animal's teeth should be
cleaned at least once daily at
home with a soft toothbrush or a
washcloth. There is evidence that
feeding commercial dry pet food
may decrease the incidence of
gingival disease.

✱ 14. Animal needs an
antibiotic shot
(long - act.
Benzathine)
(Penicillin)

Bibliography

Black AP, Crichlow RT, Saunder JR: Bacteremia during ultrasonic teeth cleaning and
extraction in the dog. JAAHA 16(4):611–616, 1980

Colmery B: Personal communication, 1982

Frost P: Canine Dentistry—A Compendium. Day Communications, 1982

Harvey CE: Veterinary Dentistry. Philadelphia, WB Saunders, 1985

Hribernik G: Dentistry for the veterinary technician, Part I. Comp Contin Educ for AHT
2(5):241–246, 1981

Hribernik G: Dentistry for the veterinary technician, Part II. The Animal Health Technician 3(2):90–96, 1982

Midwest Veterinary Advisory Board: Technique Sheets #1, 2, 5. Veterinary Products Group of American Midwest, 901 W. Oakton Street, Des Plaines, IL 60018

Stedman's Medical Dictionary, 21st ed. Baltimore, Williams & Wilkins, 1966

Studer E: The role of dry foods in maintaining healthy teeth and gums in the cat. Small Animal Clin 68(10):1124–1126, 1973

Tholen MA: Veterinary periodontal therapy. VM/SAC 77(7):1045–1053, 1982

Chapter 20

NASOPHARYNGEAL PROCEDURES

The secret of care of the patient is caring for the patient.

FRANCIS WELD PEABODY

Purpose

To obtain and examine thoroughly specimens from the upper respiratory tract

Specific Indications

1. Epistaxis
2. Nasal discharge
3. Nasal obstruction
4. Stertor
5. Upper respiratory stridor
6. Dyspnea
7. Dysphagia

Possible Complications

1. Severe epistaxis
2. Aspiration of fluid into lower airways
2. Penetration of the cribriform plate

Equipment

- Otoscope (with multiple specula) or rhinoscope
- Sterile cotton-tipped applicators
- 3.5 F polyethylene catheter
- Laryngoscope

- Dental mirror and light source
- 10 F polyethylene catheter
- Sterile saline
- Endotracheal tube
- Collection receptacle

Positioning and Restraint

General anesthesia is required for thorough examination of the nasal passages and pharynx. In our experience, no combination of sedatives or tranquilizers provides an adequate degree of immobilization or analgesia. In fact, a deep plane of anesthesia usually is required for invasive procedures involving the nasal passages.

Preparation

Because the procedures described below represent only part of a diagnostic plan for a variety of respiratory disorders (see Indications), they should be performed only after careful evaluation of historical and physical findings. We strongly suggest that high-detail survey radiographs of the nasal passages and frontal sinuses be completed before proceeding to these invasive procedures.

If a nasal biopsy is anticipated, we recommend evaluation of coagulation by performing an activated clotting time (see Chap. 31). To prevent aspiration of fluid from the nasal passages or pharynx into the lower respiratory tract, three precautions should be taken: 1) insert an appropriate-sized endotracheal tube with inflatable cuff to prevent flow of secretions down the trachea; 2) pack the nasopharynx with moistened gauze sponges to prevent caudal flow of fluid from the nasal passages; and 3) place the animal on a slightly inclined table with the head down to permit gravity flow of fluids out of the nares and mouth.

PHARYNGEAL EXAMINATION

The pharyngeal examination may be performed before or after the nasal specimen collection procedures described above. It usually is best to perform the pharyngeal examination before trauma associated with pharyngeal packing can occur.

Procedure

Technical Action
1. After placing endotracheal tube, inspect tonsils and palatine pillars carefully.

Rationale/Amplification
1. These areas may contain primary or metastatic oral neoplasms or show acute inflammation.

Technical Action

2. Palpate dorsal pharynx with gloved finger (Fig. 20-1).
3. Inspect the internal nares, using dental mirror and light source (Fig. 20-2). If necessary, retract the soft palate rostrally, using Babcock intestinal forceps.
4. Remove endotracheal tube after partial deflation of its cuff.

Rationale/Amplification

2. Enlarged lymph nodes may be discovered.
3. Posterior nasal masses may be identified.

4. Do not deflate the cuff completely, and remove the tube gently to retrieve any fluid that has entered the airway.

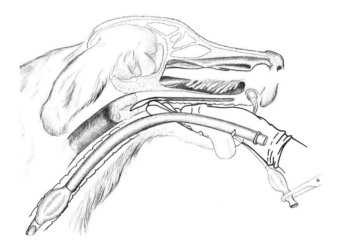

Figure 20-1   Palpating dorsal pharynx.

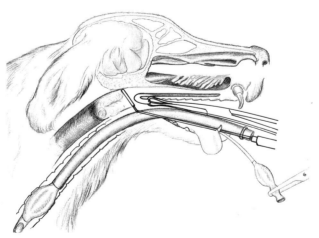

Figure 20-2   Inspecting internal nares using dental mirror.

Technical Action

5. Note larynx and epiglottis and their relationships to tongue and soft palate.

6. Note any asymmetry in the following:
   • Glottis
   • Arytenoid cartilages
   • Vocal folds
   • Laryngeal saccules
   • Aryepiglottic folds

7. Observe swallowing as animal recovers from anesthesia.

8. If abnormalities are observed and biopsy is needed or a nasal examination is to be performed, replace endotracheal tube to regain adequate plane of anesthesia.

Rationale/Amplification

5. The epiglottis should just touch the soft palate.

8. If soiled with blood or exudates, the tube should be rinsed thoroughly.

NASAL SPECIMEN COLLECTION

Procedure

Technical Action

1. Clean and disinfect external nares.

2. Pass sterile cotton-tipped applicator stick (culture swab) carefully through one external naris, and advance it caudally until it contacts firm surface.

3. Rotate swab and move it laterally and medially; then withdraw and submit specimen for culture (Fig. 20-3).

4. Advance 3.5 F catheter similarly to passage of culture swab.

Rationale/Amplification

1. Disinfection minimizes the chance of external contaminants altering culture results.

2. The swab should never be advanced a distance greater than that from the rostrum to the medial canthus. Directing it medially at first will facilitate its passage through the naris.

3. The procedure may be performed on one or both sides. If cytology is desired, a second swab is used and smears are made.
   If little or no material is obtained by the swab technique, a nasal flush is performed.

4. Again, avoid passing the catheter too far.

Technical Action

5. Attach syringe filled with 10 to 20 ml of sterile saline; inject saline slowly, moving catheter in and out during injection (Fig. 20-4).

Rationale/Amplification

5. Particulate matter and exudates are dislodged by this action.

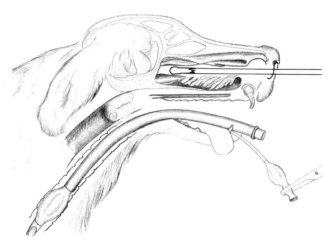

Figure 20-3 Obtaining specimen from nasal passages, using a cotton swab.

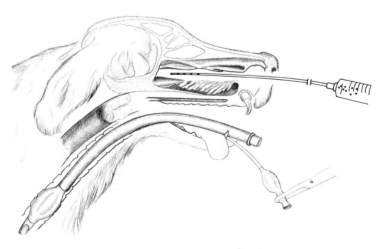

Figure 20-4 Performing nasal flush.

Technical Action

Rationale/Amplification

6. Collect effluent in sterile receptacle such as a pan or beaker.

6. The fluid is then centrifuged and the sediment is examined cytologically.
When flushing yields few or no cells for evaluation, a nasal biopsy may be performed.

NOTE: *The following steps are recommended only when a mass lesion is identified by examination or radiographs. Nasal biopsy is very traumatic and is not appropriate for diffuse nasal disease.*

7. Prepare 10 F polyethylene catheter as follows:
   • Cut end at sharp bevel with scalpel blade.
   • Make mark on catheter to indicate maximal depth of penetration.
   • Attach 20-ml syringe containing 10 ml sterile saline.

7. The bevel provides a cutting edge for the catheter.
The location of the mark is determined by measuring the distance from the rostrum to the medial canthus.

8. Place pan or beaker covered with sterile gauze below nares to collect effluent material.

8. The gauze acts as a filter for large particles.

9. Advance catheter through naris until it contacts a firm structure.

9. Do not advance farther than the premeasurement mark. It is possible to penetrate the cribriform plate and damage the meninges or brain.

10. Force the catheter in and out of the nasal passages approximately 1 to 2 cm per stroke, repeating 5 to 10 strokes (Fig. 20-5).

10. During each stroke, the syringe plunger is advanced or retracted alternately so as to produce both flushing and suction actions. Considerable bleeding frequently is encountered but usually will stop spontaneously within 5 to 10 minutes.

11. Withdraw catheter and eject syringe and catheter lumen contents through the gauze (Fig. 20-6).

12. Transfer particulate material caught in gauze mesh to slides or fixative for evaluation.

12. Large pieces of tissue may be collected for cytology and histopathology by this method.

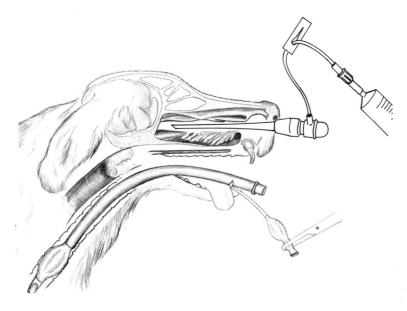

Figure 20-5 Performing nasal biopsy with altered polyethylene catheter.

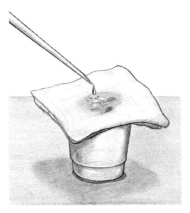

Figure 20-6 Catching particulate matter from nasal biopsy in gauze sponge.

Postbiopsy Considerations

Considerable hemorrhage may occur following nasal biopsy. If bleeding continues for more than 5 to 10 minutes, pack the nasal passages firmly with ribbon gauze. Remove nose packs before animal's recovery from anesthesia.

Bibliography

Withrow SJ: Diagnostic and therapeutic nasal flush in small animals. JAAHA 13:704–707, 1977

Withrow SJ, Susaneck SJ, Macy DW, Sheetz J: Aspiration and punch biopsy techniques for nasal tumors. JAAHA 21:551–554, 1985

Chapter 21

TRANSTRACHEAL ASPIRATION

You cannot command success, you can only deserve it.

OG MANDINO

Rd. for mon.

 Transtracheal aspiration is a diagnostic and occasionally therapeutic procedure involving the placement of a fine catheter through the cricothyroid membrane or interannular membrane of the trachea.

Purposes

1. To obtain an uncontaminated sputum sample for microbiologic and cytologic studies
2. To promote coughing in an animal with viscous respiratory secretions
3. To permit instillation of oxygen or drugs into larger lower airways

Good For Kennel Cough

Specific Indications

1. Chronic cough
2. Productive cough
3. Bronchial and peribronchial radiographic densities

Possible Complications

1. Tracheal laceration and hemorrhage
2. Acute dyspnea — difficulty breathing
3. Subcutaneous emphysema — air under skin cavity
4. Pneumomediastinum — air induced into chest who. the
5. Iatrogenic infection — infection induced organs. from procedure (man-made)

Pneumonia

mediastinum = area btw. the chest cavity + the organs.

187

Equipment Needed

- 14- to 18-gauge, 12-inch long, through-the-needle intravenous catheter (Fig. 21-1)
- 10-ml or 20-ml syringe filled with sterile physiologic saline solution
- Antiseptic soap and solution
- Local anesthetic (e.g. 2% lidocaine)
- Sterile gloves

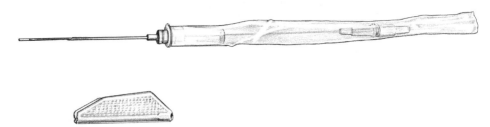

Figure 21-1   Through-the-needle catheter used for transtracheal aspiration.

Restraint and Positioning

Physical restraint is usually adequate. Some animals require tranquilization but local anesthesia is usually not necessary. General anesthesia is contraindicated because the cough reflex is suppressed. The animal is allowed to sit or to lie in sternal recumbency.

Procedure

Technical Action	Rationale/Amplification
1. Extend animal's neck so that nares point toward ceiling.	1. This position facilitates palpation and observation of the ventral aspects of the larynx and trachea.
2. Prepare skin over cricothyroid membrane or trachea by clipping hair and scrubbing skin in routine manner.	2. The cricothyroid membrane is relatively avascular and readily identifiable. This site permits easy access to the tracheal lumen and minimizes trauma to the dorsal tracheal membrane.

NOTE: *It is often advisable to use an interannular space near the thoracic inlet to permit passage of the catheter into the carina. Alternatively a long polyethylene catheter may be introduced through a separate large gauge needle inserted into the cricothyroid membrane.*

Technical Action

3. Insert needle into tracheal lumen by puncturing cricothyroid or interannular membrane at a 45-degree angle (Fig. 21-2).
4. Advance catheter to its full length (Fig. 21-3).
5. Withdraw needle from the trachea, leaving catheter in place (Fig. 21-4).
6. Rapidly infuse sterile saline (3 to 10 ml) through catheter (Fig. 21-5).
7. While animal is coughing, aspirate secretions and exudates into syringe (Fig. 21-6).

Rationale/Amplification

4. Catheter is advanced within the plastic sheath.
5. A needle guard is secured to prevent severing the catheter inadvertently.
6. The saline loosens secretion and promotes coughing.
7. Do not expect to retrieve all of the infused saline—20% or less of the infused volume is a common yield.

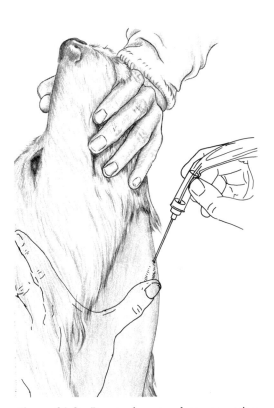

Figure 21-2 Puncturing trachea or cricothyroid membrane.

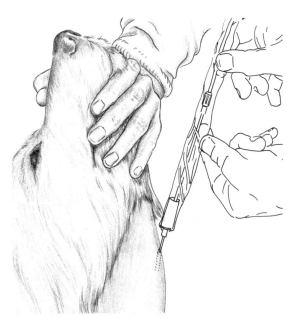

Figure 21-3 Threading catheter through needle into tracheal lumen.

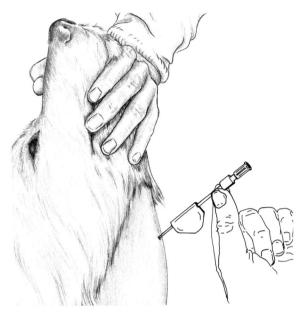

Figure 21-4 Withdrawal of needle from tracheal lumen and attachment of needle guard.

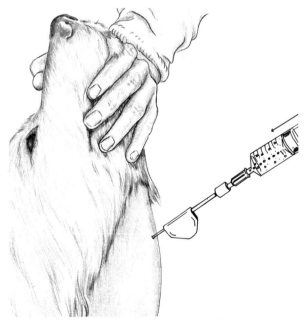

Figure 21-5 Infusing sterile saline through catheter.

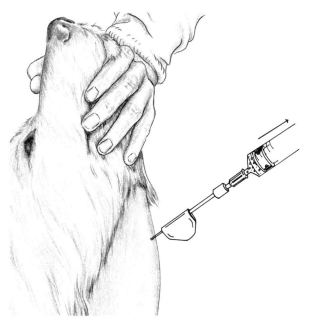

Figure 21-6 Aspirating tracheal fluids through catheter.

Technical Action	Rationale/Amplification
8. Remove catheter and apply digital pressure to puncture site for 30 seconds.	8. Pressure over the site may prevent excessive bleeding or subcutaneous or mediastinal emphysema.
9. Transfer contents of syringe to specimen tubes, and submit for culture and antimicrobial sensitivity and for cytologic examination.	✳9. Transtracheal aspiration permits sampling from the respiratory tract without contamination from the oropharynx. (mouth)
✳10. Observe patient closely for dyspnea for 30 minutes after catheter removal.	✳10. If the patient becomes markedly more dyspneic, administer oxygen.

Bibliography

Creighton SR, Wilkins RJ: Transtracheal aspiration biopsy: Technique and cytology evaluation. JAAHA 10:219–226, 1974

Rebar AH: Handbook of Veterinary Cytology. St Louis, Purina Company, 1981

Chapter 22

CENTESIS

They are able who think they are able.

VIRGIL

Centesis is a diagnostic and therapeutic procedure involving introduction of a cannula into a body cavity for the purpose of removing fluid or gas.

Purposes

1. To relieve clinical signs caused by free air or fluid in a body cavity
2. To obtain material for cytologic and/or microbiologic examination

PRINCIPLES AND TYPES OF CENTESIS

Thoracentesis

Specific Indications

1. Pleural effusion
2. Tension pneumothorax

Complications

1. Iatrogenic lung laceration and pneumothorax
2. Exacerbation of dyspnea due to restraint

Site

The site for thoracentesis varies and depends on the amount and location of pleural fluid or gas. The cannula should be introduced at the cranial edge of a rib to avoid laceration of intercostal vessels (Fig. 22-1).

Restraint and Positioning

Minimal restraint is required in most cases. Excessive use of physical or chemical restraint should be avoided. The procedure may be completed with the animal standing, sitting, or in sternal or lateral recumbency. Lateral recumbency is the most effective and safest position when pneumothorax is present, whereas the other positions are better choices when fluid is present in the pleural cavity.

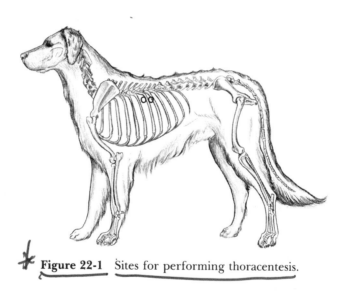

Figure 22-1 Sites for performing thoracentesis.

Pericardiocentesis

Specific Indication

Pericardial effusion

Complications

1. Laceration of myocardium
2. Laceration of lung and pneumothorax

Site

Between the fourth and sixth intercostal spaces of the left hemithorax, slightly below the costochondral junction (Fig. 22-2)

Restraint and Positioning

Minimal restraint is required. The animal is positioned in right lateral recumbency.

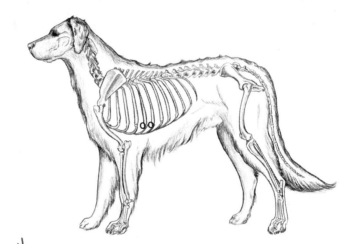

Figure 22-2 Sites for performing pericardiocentesis.

Abdominocentesis

Specific Indications

1. Abdominal trauma
2. Peritoneal effusion

Complications

1. Perforation of a hollow viscus
2. Laceration of abdominal organs
3. Peritonitis, iatrogenic

Site

The site for abdominocentesis is slightly caudal and lateral to the umbilicus (Fig. 22-3).

Restraint and Positioning

The most efficacious and convenient positions are lateral recumbency or standing positions; however, any position that is comfortable for the animal and allows pooling of fluid to the operative site is satisfactory.

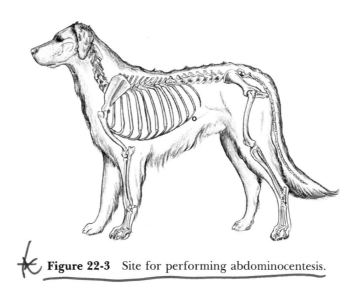

Figure 22-3 Site for performing abdominocentesis.

Cystocentesis

Specific Indications

1. Hematuria, dysuria, pyuria
2. Distention of the urinary bladder (when lower urinary tract obstruction cannot be relieved by urethral catheterization)

Complications

1. Rupture of bladder, resulting in urine leakage and possible peritonitis
2. Minimal hemorrhage, resulting in contamination of urine by blood

Site

The ventral abdomen just cranial to the pubis is the appropriate site for cystocentesis, even if the bladder can be palpated more cranially (Fig. 22-4).

Restraint and Positioning

The animal is placed in dorsal recumbency, or in lateral recumbency with the upper leg abducted to expose the inguinal area.

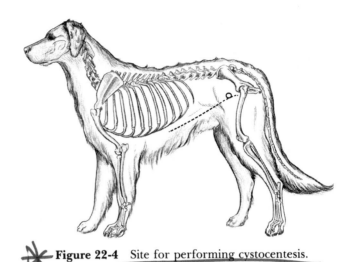

Figure 22-4 Site for performing cystocentesis.

Arthrocentesis

Specific Indications

1. Joint pain
2. Joint distention

Complications

1. Cartilage damage
2. Infectious arthritis, iatrogenic
3. Hemarthrosis, iatrogenic

Sites

The preferred sites for arthrocentesis are depicted in Figure 22-5. In each site, carefully avoid superficial blood vessels.

Restraint and Positioning

Because of the possibility of cartilage damage and the discomfort involved, sedation or general anesthesia is recommended.

Equipment Needed

- 22-gauge hypodermic needles (1″ and 3½″)
- 3-, 6-, or 12-ml syringe
- Three-way stopcock
- Fluid infusion extension tube

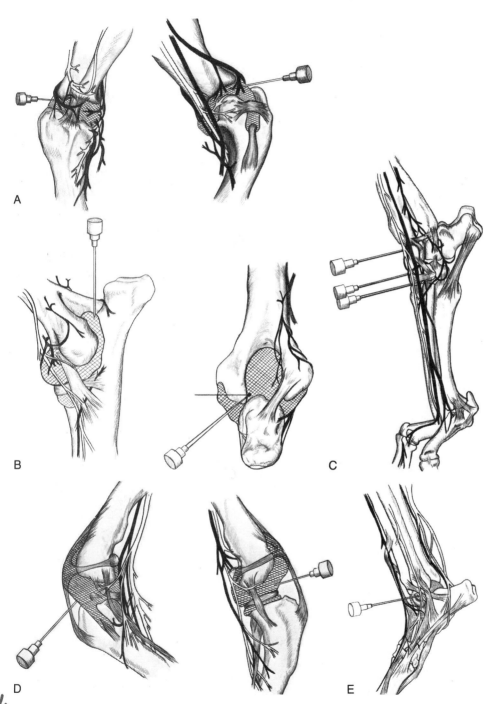

Figure 22-5 Sites for performing arthrocentesis: (*A*) shoulder, (*B*) elbow, (*C*) carpus, (*D*) stifle, and (*E*) tarsus.

CENTESIS

Procedure

Technical Action

1. Clip and prepare the operative site for aseptic surgery.

2. Palpate operative site and instill local anesthetic when indicated.

3. Penetrate skin, subcutaneous tissue and body cavity with one quick motion of sharp needle.

4. Remove fluid or air by partial withdrawal of syringe plunger.

5. Withdraw needle and syringe quickly after releasing negative pressure.

6. Transfer sample to specimen containers immediately.

Rationale/Amplification

1. See Chap. 16, pp. 141–142. Appropriate prophylaxis of contamination and infection is extremely important.

2. Local anesthesia is recommended for thoracentesis and pericardiocentesis; general anesthesia is recommended for arthrocentesis.

3. The needle is attached to an appropriate collection system. For diagnostic purposes, a 3-ml to 10-ml syringe will suffice; for therapeutic purposes, a three-way stopcock, infusion extension tube, and a 50-ml syringe are recommended.

4. If no fluid or air is obtained, the animal or limb may be moved slightly. If major repositioning is required, the needle should be withdrawn and a second puncture performed.

plunger down

6. If fluid is blood tinged, place an aliquot in a tube containing an anticoagulant.

Bibliography

Crowe DT: Diagnostic abdominal paracentesis techniques: Clinical evaluation in 129 dogs and cats. JAAHA 20:223–230, 1984

Ettinger SJ: Pericardiocentesis. Vet Clin N Amer 4:403–412, 1974

Hardy RM, Wallace LJ: Arthrocentesis and synovial membrane biopsy. Vet Clin N Amer 4:449–462, 1974

Schall WD: Thoracentesis. Vet Clin N Amer 4:395–401, 1974

Scott RC, Wilkins RJ, Greene RW: Abdominal paracentesis and cystocentesis. Vet Clin N Amer 4:413–418, 1974

Chapter 23

PERITONEAL CATHETERIZATION AND LAVAGE

An old error is always more popular than a new truth.

GERMAN PROVERB

 Peritoneal catheterization and lavage involves infusion and recovery of fluids from the peritoneal cavity for diagnostic or therapeutic purposes.

Purposes

1. To obtain fluid for diagnosis of intra-abdominal disease or injury
2. To infuse or drain medications or fluids into or out of the peritoneal cavity

Specific Indications

1. Peritoneal dialysis for renal failure
2. Acute pancreatitis
3. Urinary tract rupture
4. Ascites

Complications

1. Catheter incarceration/plugging
2. Puncture of viscus, especially urinary bladder
3. Subcutaneous infusion/leakage of fluids
4. Wound contamination/infection

Equipment Needed

- Peritoneal catheter set (Fig. 23-1)
- Infusion set or large syringe
- Scalpel blades, No. 11
- Peritoneal dialysate solutions
- Bandaging materials, including gauze and tape

Restraint and Positioning

Before performing peritoneal catheterization, allow animal to urinate, or empty bladder by urethral catheterization. In most animals local anesthesia is sufficient. A reversible narcotic sedative may be used if necessary. Place the animal in right or left lateral recumbency.

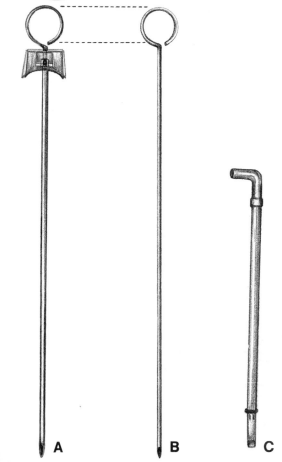

Figure 23-1   Peritoneal catheter set: (*A*) catheter with trocar/stylet in place, (*B*) trocar/stylet, and (*C*) elbow adapter and extender.

PERITONEAL CATHETERIZATION

Procedure

Technical Action

1. Clip hair from the periumbilical area of the ventral abdomen.
2. Prepare skin for aseptic surgery.
3. Make 6-mm to 8-mm incision approximately 1 cm posterior to the umbilicus.
4. Drive trocar and catheter through subcutis, abdominal muscles, and peritoneum (Fig. 23-2).

5. Direct catheter caudally.
6. Retract trocar point into catheter and advance catheter several inches into abdomen.
7. Advance remainder of catheter over the trocar/stylet in place (Fig. 23-3).

Rationale/Amplification

1. The area of catheter entry is the midline or paramedian region.
2. See Chap. 16, pp. 141–142.
3. The incision is made either in the ventral midline or slightly paramedian.
4. Back and forth rotation and a steady thrust are recommended. A popping sensation usually is felt when the trocar penetrates the peritoneum.

7. The trocar/stylet acts as a guide or director to ensure proper catheter advancement.

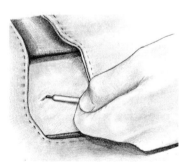

Figure 23-2 Driving trocar and catheter through abdominal wall.

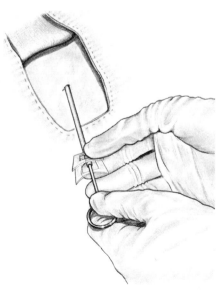

Figure 23-3 Advancing catheter into abdomen.

Technical Action

8. Attach elbow adapter and extender to end of catheter (Fig. 23-4).

Rationale/Amplification

8. Secure the attachment by wrapping with tape.

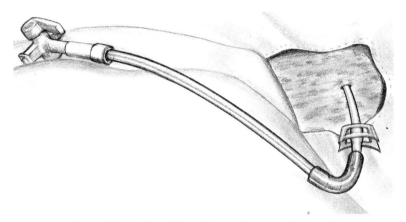

Figure 23-4 Attaching elbow adapter and extender.

Technical Action

9. If catheter apparatus does not have securing wings, apply tape to distal end of catheter, producing a wing on either side of shaft.
10. Place mattress suture through each wing and through skin (Fig. 23-5).
11. Apply antibiotic ointment to skin at point of catheter entry.
12. Carefully bandage entire abdomen with gauze and tape or elastic adhesive (Fig. 23-6).

Rationale/Amplification

10. Suturing the catheter to skin prevents unwanted traction on and migration of the catheter.
11. Prevention of infection is facilitated by this precaution.
12. Wrap the extender in gauze so that its distal end is immobile and accessible.

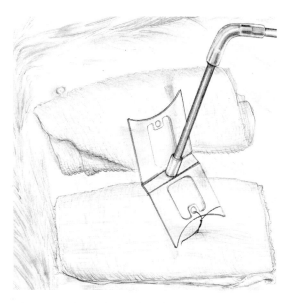

Figure 23-5 Peritoneal catheter sutured to skin.

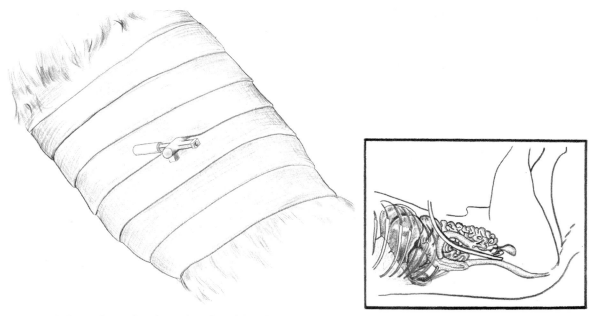

Figure 23-6 Peritoneal catheter bandaged in place.

PERITONEAL LAVAGE

Procedure

Technical Action	Rationale/Amplification
1. Attach large syringe or infusion set to catheter extender. Drain any fluid from abdomen by aspiration or gravity flow. Collect aliquot for fluid analysis, if indicated.	1. Gentle pressure on the abdomen may help in evacuating fluid.
2. Infuse approximately 30 to 50 ml dialysate solution/kg of body weight.	2. The abdomen should distend slightly but need not become taut.
3. Jostle abdomen gently with one hand and mix peritoneal cavity contents by rocking animal back and forth.	✳ 3. Leave the dialysate in the abdomen for at least 45 minutes to ensure complete osmotic exchange across the peritoneal membrane.
4. Drain fluid from abdomen by gravity flow.	4. Vigorous suction should not be used because it may result in clogging of the catheter by omentum or mesentery.
5. Repeat Nos. 1 to 4 as frequently as indicated.	5. Repeated or continuous replacements are required for peritoneal dialysis. Single or occasional infusions are used for pancreatitis or peritonitis.
6. Infuse antibacterial solutions through catheter, when indicated.	6. This treatment may be a useful adjunct to systemic therapy for acute pancreatitis or localized peritonitis.
7. If catheter is left in place but not used for infusion or drainage, flush every 4 hours with heparinized saline.	✳ 7. Fibrin clots may occlude the many openings in the end of the catheter.
8. Remove or replace catheter after 3 or 4 days.	8. Removal involves cutting the bandage and sutures and withdrawal of the catheter by gentle, steady traction. The short skin incision usually is not sutured, but the abdomen should be bandaged with a sterile dressing for 24 to 48 hours.

Bibliography

Crowe DT, Crane SW: Diagnostic abdominal paracentesis and lavage in the evaluation of abdominal injuries in dogs and cats: Clinical and experimental investigations. JAVMA 168:700–705, 1976

Kolata RJ: Diagnostic abdominal paracentesis and lavage: Experimental and clinical evaluations in the dog. JAVMA 168:697–699, 1976

Parks J, Gahring D, Greene RW: Peritoneal lavage for peritonitis and pancreatitis in twenty-two dogs. JAAHA 9:442–446, 1973

Chapter 24

VISCERAL CORE BIOPSIES (CLOSED TECHNIQUES)

The largest room of all is the room for improvement.

WALTER MACKEY

Visceral core biopsies are procedures for obtaining specimens from viscera and tissues in order to establish a histologic and/or cytologic diagnosis.

> NOTE: *Although only one technique is shown for each biopsy procedure, each needle shown can be used effectively in other viscera. Those shown represent the authors' favored technique for most cases. Because serious hemorrhage may result, an activated clotting time should be performed before proceeding (see Chap. 31). If this value is abnormal, delay procedure until normal.*

Several techniques for transthoracic pulmonary biopsy have been described in the last decade. Because the authors have limited experience with these techniques, no preferred method is described in this chapter. Please see the original articles cited in the bibliography. Precautions and risks of these procedures are worthy of your careful attention.

PLEURAL BIOPSY

Pleural biopsy is a procedure for establishing a histologic diagnosis in patients with pleural thickening or effusion.

Specific Indications

1. Confirmation of cytologic diagnosis of
   Mesothelioma
   Metastatic cancer
   Chronic pleuritis
2. Pleural thickening

Complications

1. Laceration of lung resulting in pneumothorax or hemorrhage
2. Chest wall puncture resulting in pneumothorax or hemorrhage

Equipment Needed

- Punch biopsy instrument with hook needle (Cope needle; Fig. 24-1)
- Local anesthetic (*e.g.,* 2% lidocaine)
- Skin preparation materials
- Sterile gloves

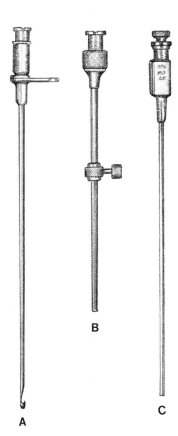

Figure 24-1 Cope needle for pleural biopsy: (*A*) obturator (with hook), (*B*) cannula, and (*C*) stylet.

Biopsy Site

Choice of site is determined by radiographic localization of areas of pleural thickening. If possible, avoid the cardiac apex/notch area.

Restraint and Positioning

Most animals require some sedation. Cooperative patients may be biopsied using local anesthesia only. Choice of chemical restraint measures should be based on the degree of respiratory insufficiency.

To maximize the space between visceral and parietal pleura, the animal should be positioned so that the biopsy site is uppermost (*e.g.*, mass next to the middle of the right eighth rib, with animal positioned in left lateral recumbency).

Procedure

Technical Action	Rationale/Amplification
1. After identifying site for biopsy, clip hair and cleanse skin.	1. See Chap. 16, pp. 141–142.
2. Make a small incision with scalpel blade.	2. Incising the skin facilitates insertion of the biopsy needle.
3. Advance biopsy needle (with stylet in place) through the incision and intercostal muscles.	
4. Before entering thorax, remove stylet from the cannula and attach syringe.	4. The needle should enter the thorax near the cranial border of a rib to avoid damaging the intercostal vessels.
5. Slowly advance needle with twisting motion until pleural cavity is entered.	5. Entry into the pleural space is detected by a sudden change in resistance.
6. Aspirate fluid and retract needle just far enough to prevent further fluid aspiration.	6. The cannula is now positioned just outside the pleural cavity.
7. Detach syringe and insert hooked obturator through outer cannula.	7. The hook opening is directed dorsally to avoid vessel damage.
8. Again, advance instrument into pleural space while applying pressure in direction of hook opening (Fig. 24-2*A*).	
9. Slowly withdraw obturator and cannula in unison until hook catches in parietal pleura (Fig. 24-2*B*).	

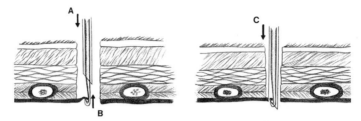

Figure 24-2 Obtaining a pleural biopsy using a Cope needle: (*A*) Advance obturator while applying lateral pressure. (*B*) Withdraw obturator until hook catches in parietal pleura. (*C*) Advance outer cannula into pleura cavity while maintaining light traction on obturator.

Technical Action	Rationale/Amplification
10. While applying slight traction on obturator, again advance outer cannula, using a rotating motion (Fig. 24-2*C*).	10. The sharpened edge of the outer cannula cuts off the specimen held within the hook.
11. Remove instrument from chest and transfer specimen to desired fixative.	
12. Repeat procedure using same skin incision.	12. Direct the hook opening ventrally during the second procedure.

Postoperative Care

Hemorrhage is usually readily controlled by digital pressure. The animal should be observed for 24 hours after biopsy to ensure early detection of pneumothorax. A follow-up radiograph often is indicated.

PERCUTANEOUS LIVER BIOPSY

Percutaneous liver biopsy is a diagnostic technique for establishing a histologic diagnosis in patients with suspected diffuse hepatic disease.

Specific Indications

1. Hepatomegaly
2. Hepatic dysfunction (*e.g.*, hypoalbuminemia, increased BSP retention, icterus, persistently elevated serum liver enzyme activities)

Contraindications

1. Abnormal hemostasis
2. Severe circulatory disturbances
3. Extrahepatic biliary obstruction
4. Small liver

Complications

1. Laceration/hemorrhage of viscera, including liver, spleen, stomach, intestine, pancreas, lung, and heart
2. Puncture of gallbladder/bile peritonitis
3. Iatrogenic infectious peritonitis

Equipment

- Menghini needle (Fig. 24-3)
- Sterile saline
- 10-ml to 12-ml syringe
- Local anesthetic (*e.g.*, 2% lidocaine)
- Sterile gloves

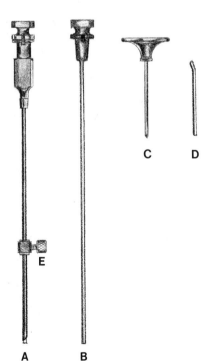

Figure 24-3 Menghini biopsy needle and accessories: (*A*) entire instrument assembled with stylet in place, (*B*) stylet, (*C*) trocar, (*D*) blocking pin, and (*E*) adjustable depth nut.

Biopsy Site/Positioning

If the liver is not palpable, the size and position of the liver should be confirmed by survey abdominal radiographs. Success of percutaneous liver biopsy depends on adequate localization of the liver. Careful direction of the needle is essential; a "hit-or-miss" approach usually is unsuccessful and is associated with marked danger of complications. A transabdominal approach is preferred when the liver is palpable beyond the costal arch; a transthoracic approach usually is preferred when the liver is normal in size.

Transabdominal percutaneous liver biopsy

Place the patient in dorsal or left-lateral recumbency. Introduce the biopsy needle through the ventral abdominal wall between the xiphoid process and the right costal arch. Advance the needle craniodorsally at an angle approximately 30 degrees right of the midsagittal plane.

Transthoracic percutaneous liver biopsy

Position the patient in sternal recumbency. Insert the needle through the thoracic wall in the seventh or eighth intercostal spaces midway between the vertebrae and sternebrae. Advance the needle slowly across the pleural space during expiration to prevent damaging the caudal lung lobe. When the diaphragm is contacted, rapidly advance the needle into the liver in a plane perpendicular to the sagittal plane.

Restraint

Sedation and local anesthesia are adequate for liver biopsy in most dogs and cats. General anesthesia may be necessary in fractious or nervous animals. Needle biopsy of the liver should not be attempted when violent or unpredictable movements prevent localization of the liver. General anesthetics that require liver metabolism or excretion should be avoided in animals with severe liver dysfunction.

Procedure

Technical Action	Rationale/Amplification
Preparatory Phase	
1. Perform activated clotting time.	**1.** See Chap. 31. If value is normal, proceed. If abnormal, delay procedure until risks have been reassessed.
2. Keep food from animal for 8 to 12 hours.	**2.** Fasting decreases stomach size and minimizes the likelihood of inadvertent puncture.
3. Give small amount of fat orally 30 to 60 minutes before biopsy.	**3.** A fatty meal may induce contraction of the gallbladder, thereby reducing its size and minimizing the chance of inadvertent puncture.

Technical Action	**Rationale/Amplification**
4. Remove ascites by abdomino-centesis.	4. Distention of the abdomen by fluid may preclude localization of the liver. See Chap. 22, pp. 194–195, 198.
5. Prepare operative site by clipping hair and cleansing and disinfecting skin in standard manner.	5. Aseptic technique should be exercised throughout the biopsy procedure. See Chap. 16, pp. 141–142.

Operative Phase

1. Inject local anesthetic into skin and parietal peritoneum or parietal pleura.	1. It is not necessary to anesthetize the liver capsule.
2. Aspirate 3 or 4 ml of sterile physiologic saline solution into 12-ml syringe.	2. Saline is used to clear debris from the biopsy needle and to expel the biopsy specimen.
3. Make 2-mm incision in skin, or use trocar to create an entry site for biopsy needle.	3. This step facilitates introduction of the blunt needle/stylet.
4. Advance needle (with stylet in place) in predetermined direction (Fig. 24-4*A*) and gently explore with needle until liver capsule is contacted (Fig. 24-4*B*).	4. Firm thrusts may be required to penetrate the peritoneum or pleura. Use the depth nut to prevent excessive penetration and damage to viscera.
5. Remove stylet and insert blocking pin (Fig. 24-4*C*). Attach syringe.	5. The blocking pin prevents aspiration of the liver specimen into the syringe.
6. With needle adjacent to liver, gently expel 0.5 to 1 ml of saline.	6. This step expels any blood or fibrin that may be occluding the needle lumen.
7. Set and secure depth nut for desired length of biopsy by measuring from skin to primary edge of depth nut (Fig. 24-4*D*)	7. The length of biopsy varies from 1 to 5 cm, depending on animal and liver size.
8. Create negative pressure by withdrawing syringe plunger.	8. This suction draws the liver to the needle. The negative pressure must be maintained throughout the procedure.
9. Rapidly thrust needle and syringe inward until nut contacts skin, and immediately withdraw entire needle (see Fig. 24-4*D*).	9. When performed properly, the liver excursion phase of the biopsy procedure takes less than 1 second. Do not wobble or rotate the needle during this cutting phase.

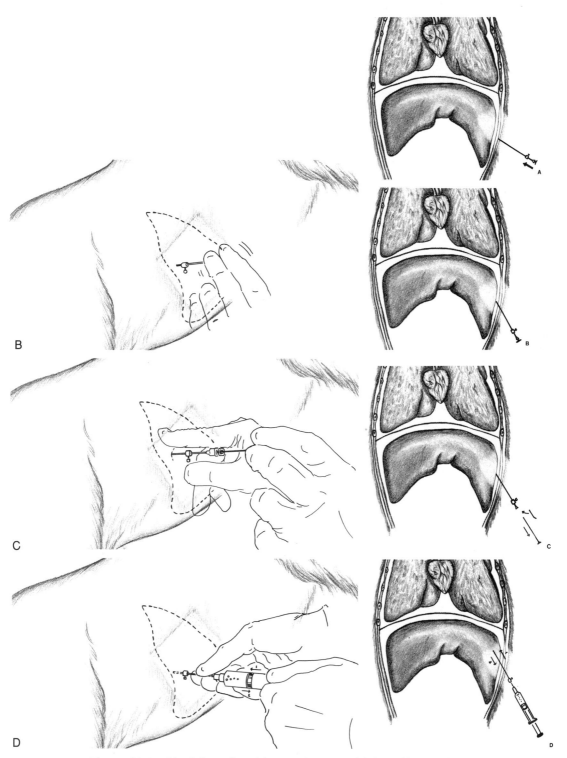

Figure 24-4 Obtaining a liver biopsy using Menghini needle: (*A*) Pierce abdominal wall with needle (stylet in place). (*B*) Advance needle with stylet in place through peritoneum and gently explore with needle until liver capsule is contacted. (*C*) Remove stylet and insert blocking pin. (*D*) Thrust needle into liver while aspirating; withdraw immediately.

Technical Action	Rationale/Amplification
10. Holding needle directly over the fixative solution, gently expel liver specimen from needle by ejecting several milliliters of saline through the needle.	**10.** Gentle handling prevents excessive fragmentation of the specimen.
11. Repeat procedure as required or indicated.	**11.** Generally at least two specimens are obtained, from slightly different locations in the liver.

Postoperative Care

Observe the patient for several hours after the procedure to determine whether excessive hemorrhage has occurred. When the specimen is heavily bile stained, particularly careful observation for signs of bile peritonitis should be emphasized to the animal's owner. Development of signs such as sudden anorexia or vomiting should be pursued vigorously in such cases.

PERCUTANEOUS KIDNEY BIOPSY

Percutaneous kidney biopsy is a procedure for establishing a histologic diagnosis in patients with unilateral or bilateral renal disease. It is particularly valuable in obtaining a specimen to predict functional recovery from renal disease.

Specific Indications

1. Chronic renal failure
2. Persistent proteinuria (suspect glomerulopathy)
3. Enlarged kidney(s)
4. Small kidney(s)
5. Irregular kidney shape

Contraindications

1. Bleeding/clotting disorders
2. Nonpalpable kidneys

Complications

1. Renal or perirenal hemorrhage
2. Retroperitoneal or intraperitoneal urine leakage

Equipment

- Vim Tru-Cut biopsy needle (Fig. 24-5)
- Scalpel blade (No. 11)
- Local anesthetic (*e.g.*, 2% lidocaine)
- Skin preparation materials
- Sterile gloves

Biopsy Site

Left or right paralumbar fossa

Restraint and Positioning

The animal is held in left or right lateral recumbency. General anesthesia rarely is required, but sedation or tranquilization often is needed.

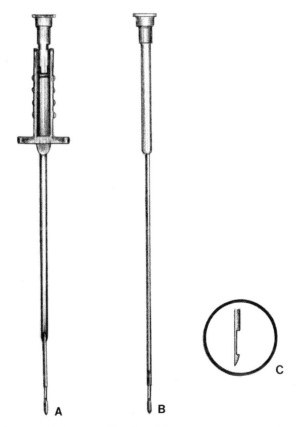

Figure 24-5   Vim Tru-Cut biopsy needle: (*A*) entire instrument assembled, (*B*) inner obturator, and (*C*) close-up side view of obturator tip.

Prebiopsy Considerations

The patient should be evaluated for coagulation abnormalities. Animals with oliguric or anuric renal failure should be treated and adequate urine production realized before biopsy. Intravenous fluids are given during the biopsy and recovery periods to prevent decreased renal perfusion.

Procedure

Technical Action	Rationale/Amplification
1. Isolate kidney to be biopsied in one hand by deep palpation.	1. If isolation is not accomplished, another biopsy technique should be used.
2. Prepare skin of paralumbar fossa overlying kidney in a routine manner; inject local anesthetic into skin at proposed biopsy site.	2. See Chap. 16, pp. 141–142.
3. Make a small stab incision with scalpel blade.	
4. Advance Vim-Tru-cut needle through incision and retroperitoneal tissue toward either pole of kidney.	
5. Introduce end of outer cannula, with inner obturator retracted, through renal capsule 1 to 2 mm, and direct it parallel or perpendicular to longitudinal axis of kidney (Fig. 24-6A).	5. The point of the needle should never be directed toward the renal pelvis because penetration of the central portion of the kidney may result in laceration of major blood vessels.
6. With handle of outer cannula held in position, advance inner obturator into kidney (Fig. 24-6B).	6. A notch in the obturator accepts the renal tissue to be removed.
7. While holding inner obturator handle, advance outer cannula into kidney (Fig. 24-6C).	7. This step cuts off the specimen and protects it within the biopsy notch of obturator.
8. Pull needle directly out of kidney and skin and pass it to an assistant.	8. The sample is transferred immediately to the appropriate fixative solution.
9. Apply firm digital pressure to biopsy site while kidney is held.	9. Pressure is applied for approximately 5 minutes.
10. *Assistant:* Advance inner obturator to expose specimen and transfer specimen to fixative immediately.	

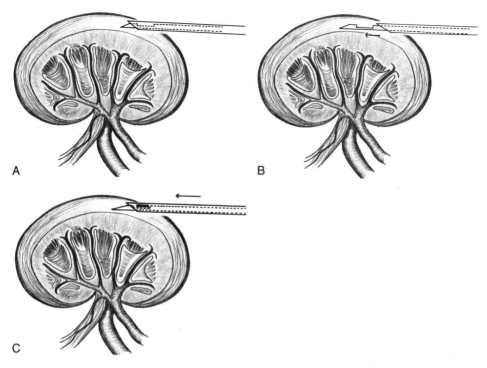

Figure 24-6 Obtaining a kidney biopsy using a Vim Tru-Cut needle: (*A*) Direct needle perpendicular or parallel to the long axis of the kidney. (*B*) Advance inner obturator. (*C*) Advance outer cannula.

Postbiopsy Considerations

Many animals have microscopic hematuria for 12 to 72 hours, whereas only a few have gross hematuria. Severe hemorrhage rarely occurs when proper technique is used.

TRANSPERINEAL PROSTATE BIOPSY

Transperineal prostate biopsy is a percutaneous method of acquiring specimens for histologic diagnosis of prostatic disease.

Specific Indications

1. Prostatomegaly
2. Prostatic deformity or asymmetry

Contraindications

1. Prostate not palpable per rectum
2. Fluctuant enlargement of the prostate
3. Bleeding/clotting disorders

Complications

1. Severe intrapelvic hemorrhage
2. Puncture or laceration of rectum, small intestine, urethra, or urinary bladder

Equipment

- Vim-Silverman biopsy needle (Fig. 24-7)
- Local anesthetic (*e.g.*, 2% lidocaine)
- Scalpel blade (No. 11)
- Skin preparation materials
- Sterile gloves

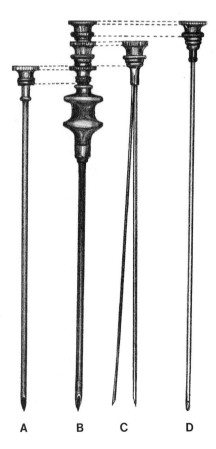

Figure 24-7 Vim-Silverman needle for visceral core biopsies: (*A*) stylet, (*B*) entire instrument assembled, (*C*) cutting prongs, and (*D*) obturator.

A   B   C   D

Biopsy Site

Needle entry is at a point on the skin equidistant between the anal orifice and tuber ischium on the desired side.

Restraint and Positioning

Because of the discomfort produced by digital rectal palpation, heavy sedation or general anesthesia is recommended. If sedation is used, local anesthesia should be added. The animal is positioned in sternal or lateral recumbency, with the tail reflected dorsolaterally.

Procedure

Technical Action

1. Clip perineal region and prepare for biopsy.

2. Inject local anesthetic in skin biopsy site, if sedation is used.
3. Make 2-mm stab incision in perineal skin with scalpel blade.
4. Place a gloved middle or index finger in rectum and secure prostate against bony pelvis by digital pressure (Fig. 24-8A).
5. Advance Vim-Silverman needle, with stylet inside cannula, cranially and parallel to ventrolateral rectal wall, until it contacts lobe of prostate (Fig. 24-8B).
6. Press needle to enter prostate approximately 1 mm. Remove stylet and slide cutting prongs and obturator into cannula until prongs just contact prostate.
7. Forcefully advance obturator 3 to 15 mm, while cannula is held in position. (Fig. 24-8C)

8. Advance cannula while obturator is held in place (Fig. 24-8D).

Rationale/Amplification

1. Special care is taken to cleanse the area because of the increased risk of fecal contamination.

4. If the prostate cannot be isolated and secured within the pelvic canal, biopsy should not be attempted.
5. Proceed slowly to avoid damaging vessels and organs.

7. The length of the biopsy specimen is governed by the size of the prostate. Do not permit the obturator to extend to the opposite pole of the prostate lobe.
8. The specimen is severed from the gland and is contained in the obturator notch.

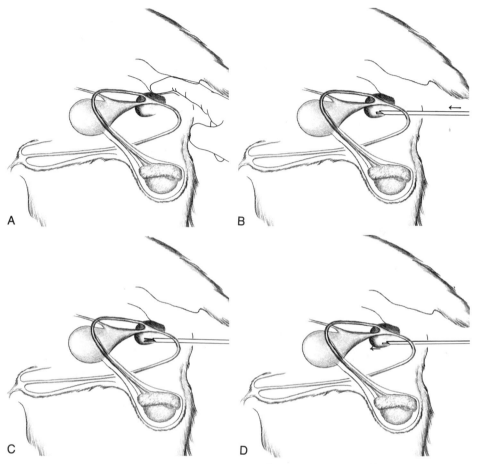

Figure 24-8 Obtaining a prostate biopsy using a Vim-Silverman needle: (*A*) Secure prostate in place by palpating per rectum. (*B*) Advance needle through perineum and parallel to rectum until prostate is contacted. (*C*) Advance inner obturator. (*D*) Advance outer cannula.

Technical Action	**Rationale/Amplification**
9. Remove entire needle assembly from prostate and perineum; immediately apply digital pressure to biopsy site per rectum.	**9.** Pressure should be maintained for at least 2 minutes.
10. Transfer specimen to culture tube or fixative immediately.	

Postbiopsy Complications

Frank hematuria may be observed for 1 to 3 days after biopsy.

Bibliography

Berquist TH et al.: Transthoracic needle biopsy. Mayo Clin Proc 55:475–481, 1980

Feldman EC, Ettinger SJ: Percutaneous transthoracic liver biopsy in the dog. JAVMA 169:805–810, 1976

Leeds EB, Leav I: Perineal punch biopsy of the canine prostate gland. JAVMA 154:925–934, 1969

McEvoy RD, Begley MD, Antic R: Percutaneous biopsy of intrapulmonary mass lesions. Cancer 51:2321–2326, 1983

Menghini G: One-second biopsy of the liver. Gastroenterology 35:190–199, 1958

Michel RP, Lushpihan A, Ahmed AN: Pathologic findings of transthoracic needle aspiration in the diagnosis of localized pulmonary lesions. Cancer 51:1663–1672, 1983

Roudebush P, Green RA, Digilio KM: Percutaneous fine-needle aspiration biopsy of the lung. JAAHA 17:109–115, 1981

Weaver AD: Transperineal punch biopsy of the canine prostate gland. J Small Anim Pract 18:573–577, 1977

Chapter 25

UROHYDROPROPULSION

Success is simply a matter of luck. Ask any failure.

EARL WILSON

Urohydropropulsion is a therapeutic procedure for removal of foreign material (*e.g.*, uroliths) from the urethra of male dogs.

Specific Indication

Lower urinary tract obstruction by uroliths

Equipment

- Sterile flexible urethral catheter
- 20- to 50-ml syringe
- Sterile physiologic saline
- Examination glove
- Lubricating jelly

Restraint and Positioning

The dog is held in lateral recumbency and the prepuce is retracted as if for urethral catheterization. The operation requires placing one finger in the rectum. Sedation or tranquilization is recommended.

Procedure

Technical Action	**Rationale/Amplification**
1. Pass a sterile flexible catheter up urethra to point of obstruction and then withdraw approximately 1 inch.	1. See Chap. 12, pp. 112–115. A large-gauge catheter should be used to ensure a tight fit.
2. Attach syringe containing 20 to 50 ml of physiologic saline to open end of catheter.	2. Lubricants such as mineral oil may be added if desired.
3. Place operator's lubricated, gloved finger in rectum and occlude lumen of pelvic urethra by applying digital pressure through ventral rectal wall.	
4. Compress the external urethral orifice around the catheter by digital pressure.	4. The lower urethra and syringe are now a closed system.
5. Inject saline rapidly until a rebound of syringe plunger occurs (Fig. 25-1).	5. The urethra will be maximally dilated at this time.

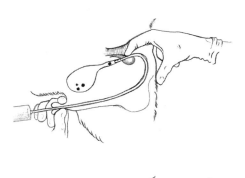

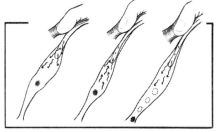

Figure 25-1 Schematic representation of forces and fluid flow during urohydropropulsion.

Technical Action	**Rationale/Amplification**
6. If the largest calculus is too large to pass by the os penis under any circumstances, the operator releases pressure on the proximal urethra. If the largest calculus may pass the os penis, the external urethral orifice pressure is released.	**6.** This sudden release of pressure causes a back flow, and the calculus moves toward the urinary bladder. The sudden release of external pressure causes flow, and the calculus moves toward the external urethral orifice.
7. If no movement of a calculus is apparent after three or four attempts, discontinue the procedure.	**7.** Sometimes, alternating the direction of urethral fluid flow will help to free a calculus. Often it is necessary to repeat this procedure several times to force a calculus back into the bladder or to cause it to be voided.

Bibliography

Osborne CA, Low DG, Finco DR: Urohydropropulsion. In Canine and Feline Urology. Philadelphia, WB Saunders, 1972

Chapter 26

PROSTATIC MASSAGE/WASHING

Only a mediocre person is always at his best.

SOMERSET MAUGHAM

Prostatic massage/washing is a procedure by which prostatic fluid is obtained.

Purposes

1. To examine prostatic secretions microscopically for microorganisms and cellular elements
2. To obtain prostatic secretions for bacteriologic culture and antibiotic sensitivity testing

Specific Indications

1. Pyuria
2. Hematuria
3. Bloody urethral discharge
4. Prostatic asymmetry
5. Prostatomegaly

Complications

1. Rupture of prostatic abscess
2. Rectal perforation
3. Ascending urinary tract infection

Equipment needed

- Equipment for urinary catheterization of male dog (See Chap. 12, pp. 110–112)
  Cotton
  Skin disinfectant or mild soap
  Sterile flexible urinary catheter of appropriate size
  Sterile gloves
- Sterile containers for two specimens
- Two 5-ml syringes, each containing 5 ml sterile saline

Restraint and Positioning

The dog is restrained in a standing position for the prostatic massage and washing. If desired, the dog can be placed in lateral recumbency while the urinary catheter is introduced. Usually two assistants are needed for this procedure.

Procedure

Technical Action	Rationale/Amplification
1. Label sterile containers for urine and prostatic fluid.	
2. Advance urinary catheter into urinary bladder and empty urine from bladder.	2. See Chap. 12, pp. 112–115. It is important to premeasure the catheter by holding it in its approximate intraurethral position near but not touching the dog.
3. Instill 5 ml of sterile saline through catheter into urinary bladder, then aspirate this saline into same syringe and place into sterile container.	3. Washing the bladder and comparing results of the prostatic massage and washing helps to identify organisms and cells that are found only in the prostate.
4. Place gloved finger in rectum.	
5. Withdraw urinary catheter so that catheter tip is in portion of urethra distal to prostate.	5. Premeasuring the catheter makes it possible to estimate the approximate location of the prostatic urethra. In some dogs, the catheter tip may be palpated as it is moved within the pelvic urethra.
6. Massage prostate with gloved finger in rectum for 1 minute (Fig. 26-1). Ask assistant to collect any fluid that comes out of catheter during massage.	6. Vigorous massage should be avoided if prostatic abscess is suspected.

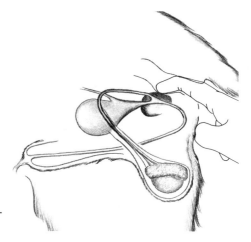

Figure 26-1 Massage of prostate per rectum.

Technical Action

7. Instill 5 ml of sterile saline through catheter into urinary bladder, then advance catheter into bladder again and aspirate this saline.
8. Place second aspirate into prostatic fluid container.
9. Submit both specimens for bacteriologic and cytologic evaluation.

Rationale/Amplification

7. Instillation of saline after the massage will enable collection of small amounts of prostatic secretions released during prostatic massage.

9. Specimens should be labeled with date, time, animal identification, and type of specimen.

NOTE: *There is evidence that accurate diagnosis of chronic bacterial prostatitis is made more readily by analysis of ejaculate than from a specimen obtained by the prostatic massage and washing procedure. This is true in particular if the dog has a concurrent urinary tract infection. (See Chap. 27 for semen collection procedure.)*

Bibliography

Barsanti JA, Finco DR: Canine bacterial prostatitis. Vet Clin N Amer 9(4):679–700, 1979

Barsanti JA, Prasse KW, Crowell WA, Shotts EB, Finco DR: Evaluation of various techniques for diagnosis of chronic bacterial prostatitis in the dog. JAVMA 183(2):219–224, 1983

Chapter 27

SEMEN COLLECTION AND ARTIFICIAL INSEMINATION

When love and skill work together, expect a masterpiece.

JOHN RUSKIN

Canine semen is collected for diagnosis of suspected prostatic disease or infertility. Artificial insemination is a technique used in place of natural breeding in fertile breeding bitches and sires.

SEMEN COLLECTION

Purposes

1. To evaluate spermatogenic capability of proposed sire as part of a prebreeding or prepurchase examination
2. To obtain specimens for culture or cytology from prostate and testicle/epididymis
3. To obtain semen for artificial insemination or freezing

Complications

1. Paraphimosis
2. Physical injury to male or handlers

Equipment

- Artificial vagina (latex rubber cone, with attached sterile graduated centrifuge tube)
- Aqueous lubricating jelly

Preparation and Restraint

The prospective sire and an estrous bitch are brought together in a quiet room. Both dogs should be restrained by leash and the floor should not be excessively slippery. The male and female may be allowed to play. The male is encouraged to sniff the vulva of the bitch. If the female resists the male's attention by snapping or biting, she should be muzzled and restrained to prevent injury to the male or the handlers. The handler of the estrous bitch should squat or kneel near the female's head and prevent her from biting the male (see Chap. 1). This is particularly important once the male starts to mount.

> NOTE: *When semen is collected for diagnostic purposes only, most males do not require a teaser bitch. A docile, anestrous bitch usually will suffice. Inexperienced or shy males may need an estrous teaser to stimulate erection and ejaculation.*

Attach the collection tube to the latex rubber cone. Lubricate the cone lightly with jelly near its broad end to facilitate removal of artificial vagina after ejaculation.

Procedure

Technical Action

1. When male is ready to mount female, semen collector kneels at male's side.

2. Place artificial vagina over end of penis and use cone to gently slide prepuce caudally, enclosing the erect penis to point proximal to bulbus glandis (Fig. 27-1)

Rationale/Amplification

1. Collection should be performed where the male is most comfortable. This is usually on the floor rather than a table.

2. Kneel next to the dog and retract the prepuce with artificial vagina held in one hand. Support the attached tube with the other hand. This is necessary to prevent swinging and resultant breakage of the tube. Once the artificial vagina is in place, the dog usually will start pelvic thrusting and ejaculation. A few drops of clear ejaculate is followed quickly by the white, sperm-laden semen.

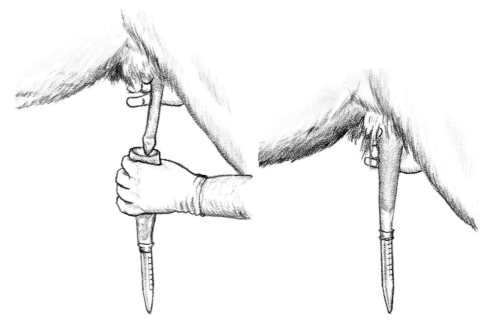

Figure 27-1 Placing artificial vagina over erect penis.

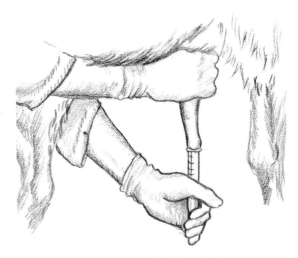

Figure 27-2 Collecting ejaculate.

Technical Action	Rationale/Amplification
3. Maintain gentle pressure on the penis, which is still ensheathed in artificial vagina. (Fig. 27-2).	**3.** This step simulates the natural tie.

Technical Action	Rationale/Amplification
4. Collect 1 to 20 ml of third fraction of ejaculate.	4. If the semen is to be used for artificial insemination, a total volume of approximately 5 ml of semen is collected. If prostatic disease is suspected, larger amounts should be collected. If breeding soundness is being tested, the last fraction, which is largely prostatic secretion, should be collected in a separate tube so as not to dilute the sperm-laden fraction.
6. After collection is complete, carefully remove artificial vagina from shaft of penis.	6. Removal may not be possible in large dogs. If artificial vagina is snug, do not attempt to remove it—let erection subside naturally. Disconnect collection tube and process semen sample.
7. Remove teaser bitch from room.	
8. Allow male to rest or walk while erection subsides.	8. Always check male after erection subsides for paraphimosis or trauma to the penis. Never send a dog home until the penis is completely retracted into the prepuce.

ARTIFICIAL INSEMINATION

Purposes

1. To prevent exposure of male to venereally transmitted diseases
2. To breed more than one bitch with one ejaculate
3. To inseminate bitch with frozen, stored semen

Specific Indications

1. Physical abnormalities of male or female that prevent natural service
2. Behavioral abnormalties of male or female that prevent natural service

Complication

Vaginal laceration

Equipment

- Insemination pipette
- Syringe
- Aqueous lubricating jelly

Preparation and Restraint

The bitch to be inseminated is restrained in a standing position. Chemical restraint measures rarely are required. The assistant holds the tail to one side to expose the perineal area (see Chap. 1).

Procedure

Technical Action

1. Clean vestibule of excess discharge with moistened cotton.
2. Slide blunt pipette (containing semen) just below dorsal commissure of vulva and through vestibule and vagina to level of cervix.

Rationale/Amplification

2. The pipette is directed craniodorsally at a 45-degree angle from a horizontal plane until it has passed through the vestibule, to avoid contacting the clitoris. Then direct it cranially in a horizontal plane.

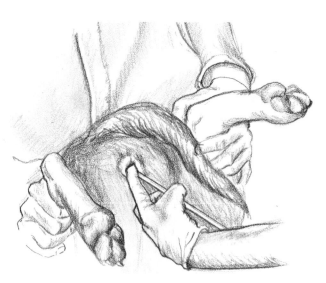

Figure 27-3 Elevating hindquarters of bitch while insemination pipette is inserted.

3. Gently eject semen from pipette, using a syringe and gravity flow.

4. Eject semen remaining in pipette by forcing 2 to 4 ml of air through it with a syringe.

5. Elevate bitch's hindquarters by grasping stifles and raising legs off floor (Fig. 27-3).

5. This position helps to retain semen at the cervix. If possible, the hindquarters should be elevated for 5 minutes.

6. Remove pipette as soon as semen is deposited.

Bibliography

Seager SWJ, Platz CC: Artificial insemination and frozen semen in the dog. Vet Clin N Amer 7:757–764, 1977

Seager SWJ, Platz CC: Collection and evaluation of canine semen. Vet Clin N Amer 7:765–773, 1977

Chapter 28

VAGINAL EXAMINATION AND SPECIMEN COLLECTION

I hear and I forget. I see and I remember. I do and I understand.

CHINESE PROVERB

Visual and digital examination of the vaginal mucosa are diagnostic methods essential to a thorough evaluation of the lower female genital tract. Samples are easily obtained for cytologic examination and microbiologic study.

Purposes

1. To ascertain the physical characteristics of the mucosal surface of the vagina by inspection and palpation
2. To obtain cytologic and microbiologic specimens from the vagina

Specific Indications

1. Vulvar or vaginal discharge
2. Attraction of males
3. Infertility
4. Dysuria
5. Tenesmus
6. Vulvar swelling
7. Estrus determination

Complications

Vaginal laceration

Equipment

- Sterile examination glove
- Vaginal speculum and light source, anoscope, or proctoscope (adult or pediatric) (Fig. 28-1)
- Sterile, guarded, cotton-tipped applicator (for microbiologic specimen)
- Cotton-tipped applicator (for cytologic specimen)
- Aqueous lubricating jelly

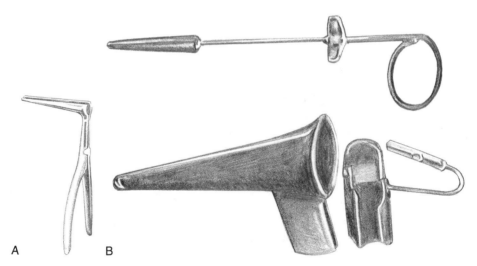

Figure 28-1   Instruments used for vaginal examination: (A) speculum, and (B) anoscope.

Restraint and Positioning

These procedures are best completed with the animal standing. The holder cradles the animal in one arm while raising the tail with the other. It may be advisable to muzzle the dog in some cases.

Preparation

If the perineum is heavily soiled, clean the perivulvar skin and hair thoroughly, using mild soap and water. Remove excess vulvar discharge with a cotton pledget.

Procedure

Technical Action	Rationale/Amplification
Specimen Collection	
1. Grasp vulva with thumb and index finger, and introduce a guarded, sterile cotton-tipped applicator stick just below dorsal vulvar commissure into vestibule and direct it along dorsal vaginal wall (Fig. 28-2).	
2. Advance swab tip out of plastic guard.	
3. Move tip from side to side or rotate it. Avoid irritating urethral papilla (orifice).	**3.** Nos. 3 and 4 ensure adequate sampling of the vaginal mucosa.
4. Move tip back and forth in cranial and caudal direction.	
5. Pull swab back into guard and remove apparatus from vagina.	
6. Immediately inoculate culture or transport media.	
7. Repeat Nos. 1, 3, and 4 with a standard cotton-tipped applicator to obtain specimen for cytologic examination.	

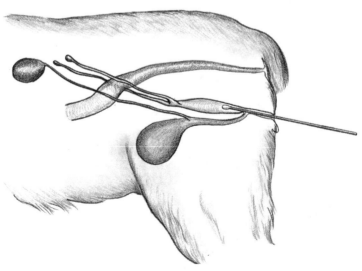

Figure 28-2 Obtaining a swab specimen of the vagina.

Technical Action

8. Remove swab and immediately roll tip across faces of two or more glass slides.

9. Allow slides to air dry and stain them immediately.

Digital Examination

1. Grasp vulva with thumb and index finger and advance gloved, lubricated index finger dorsal to clitoral fossa and into vagina (Fig. 28-3).

2. Palpate urethral papilla, vaginal wall, cervix, and pelvic bones.

3. Remove finger slowly and examine it for discharges.

Rationale/Amplification

8. Do not smear the tip on the slide—roll it!

1. Proper positioning of finger is ensured by introducing it just below the dorsal vulvar commissure and direct it at a 45-degree angle to the horizontal plane until the vagina is entered.

2. Use slow, gentle motions to avoid damage to the fragile mucous membranes.

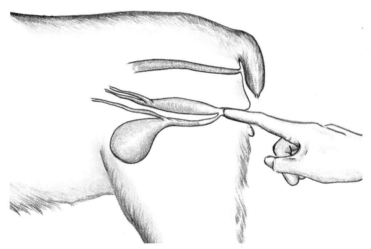

Figure 28-3 Performing digital vaginal examination.

Visual Examination

1. Grasp vulva with thumb and index finger, and introduce speculum into vestibule just below dorsal vulvar commissure. Advance instrument craniodorsally at angle approximately 45 degrees from horizontal plane until it passes through vestibule, then direct it horizontally (Fig. 28-4).

1. Be careful not to catch the speculum in the clitoral fossa because this will cause marked discomfort.

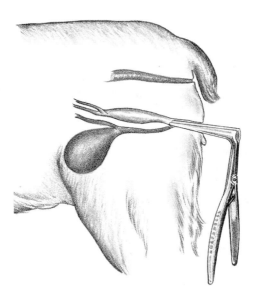

Figure 28-4 Inserting vaginal speculum.

Technical Action

2. Remove obturator, if anoscope or proctoscope is used; examine all surfaces of vaginal mucosa, proceeding from cranial to caudal. Note appearance of external urethral orifice.
3. Withdraw vaginal speculum slowly, maintaining original directional orientation.

Rationale/Amplification

2. If abnormalities are noted, a swab for cytology or culture, or a biopsy specimen, is obtained.

Bibliography

Settergren I: Examination of the canine genital system. Vet Clin North Am 1:103–118, 1971

Chapter 29

BONE MARROW ASPIRATION AND BIOPSY

Wonder rather than doubt is the root of knowledge.

ABRAHAM JOSHUA HESCHEL

Bone marrow aspiration and *biopsy* are diagnostic procedures involving the introduction of a rigid, hollow needle into the marrow-containing, cancellous part of either a long or flat bone.

Purposes

1. To identify and quantitate abnormal cell populations in bone marrow
2. To identify abnormal maturation of hematopoietic stem cell lines

Specific Indications

1. Nonregenerative anemia
2. Thrombocytopenia
3. Persistent leukopenia
4. Atypical cells in blood
5. Monoclonal dysproteinemia
6. Suspected osteomyelitis
7. Suspected nonhematopoietic neoplasia of bone
8. Clinical staging of lymphoma or mast cell tumors

Complications

1. Bleeding and hematoma formation at operative site, especially when bleeding disorders are present
2. Puncture or laceration of muscles, nerves, or blood vessels
3. Osteomyelitis (iatrogenic)

Equipment

- Bone marrow aspiration needles (Fig. 29-1)
    16-gauge Rosenthal needle or Illinois needle for medium-sized or large dogs
    18-gauge Rosenthal needle for small dogs and cats
- Jamshidi bone marrow biopsy needles (Fig. 29-2)
    12-gauge (adult) for most dogs
    14-gauge (pediatric) for small dogs and cats
- Sterile drape or towels
- Sterile gloves
- Antiseptic solutions and gauze sponges
- Local anesthetic (*e.g.,* 2% lidocaine)

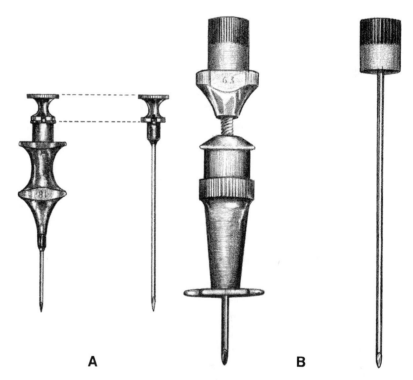

Figure 29-1 Bone marrow aspiration needles: (*A*) 18-gauge Rosenthal needle with matched stylet, and (*B*) 16-gauge Illinois needle with matched stylet and depth stop.

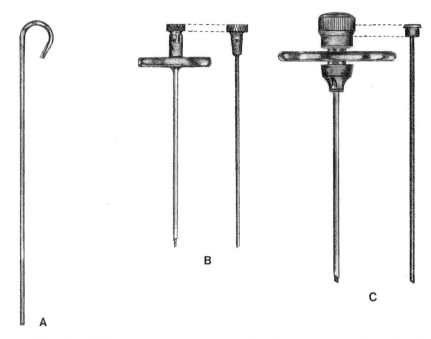

Figure 29-2 Jamshidi bone marrow biopsy needles: (*A*) specimen expeller, (*B*) pediatric, and (*C*) adult.

- Syringes
    5-ml and 20-ml
- Needles
    22- and 25-gauge
- Laboratory equipment
    Precleaned microscope slides
    Coverslips
    Culture tubes (when indicated)
- Scalpel blade (No. 11)
- Fixative (formalin or Zenker's fixative)

Procedure

Technical Action	Rationale/Amplification
Preparatory Phase	
1. Give tranquilizer, sedative, or general anesthetic as required for comfort and immobilization.	1. Most severely anemic animals do not require systemic chemical restraint. Excessive movement may result in contamination of biopsy site, laceration of tissues, or increased pain.

Technical Action	Rationale/Amplification
2. Restrain animal in appropriate position for site of aspiration or biopsy (see below and Chap. 1).	
3. Clip hair from operative site, using No. 40 clipper blade. Mark proposed entry site.	
4. Prepare skin area for aseptic surgery and drape.	**4.** See Chap. 16, pp. 141–142.

Iliac Crest Aspiration and Biopsy

Technical Action	Rationale/Amplification
Performance Phase	
1. Restrain animal in lateral recumbency.	**1.** With an unanesthetized animal, two persons may be needed for restraint to avoid contamination of the operative site.
2. Locate dorsal iliac crest and mark site for entry (Fig. 29-3A).	**2.** In the obese patient, it is frequently difficult to locate the dorsal iliac crest. Deep palpation will guide the operator.
3. Infiltrate marked area with local anesthetic in skin, subcutis, and periosteum.	**3.** The periosteum is the region of greatest sensitivity.
4. Make 3-mm stab incision in skin.	**4.** A small skin incision facilitates insertion of the large, blunt needle.

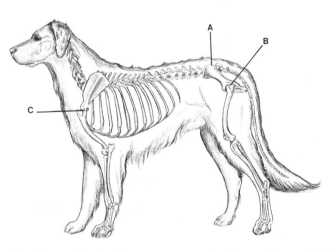

Figure 29-3   Sites for performing bone marrow aspiration or biopsy: (*A*) iliac crest, (*B*) trochanteric fossa, and (*C*) head of humerus.

Technical Action

5. Advance bone marrow needle with its stylet in place through incision.

6. Advance needle by rotation and steady pressure (Fig. 29-4*A*).

7. Aspiration technique
   a. When needle penetrates the outer cortex of bone, remove stylet.
   b. Attach 20-ml syringe and apply negative pressure by forcefully withdrawing syringe plunger (Fig. 29-4*B*).

Rationale/Amplification

5. The tip of the needle (or stylet) is brought into contact with the dorsal iliac crest and directed ventrally, parallel to a sagittal plane.

6. Avoid unnecessary wobbling by pronating and supinating forearm.

7.
   a. There is usually decreased resistance when the marrow cavity is entered.
   b. The actual aspiration usually causes considerable discomfort for the unanesthetized animal.

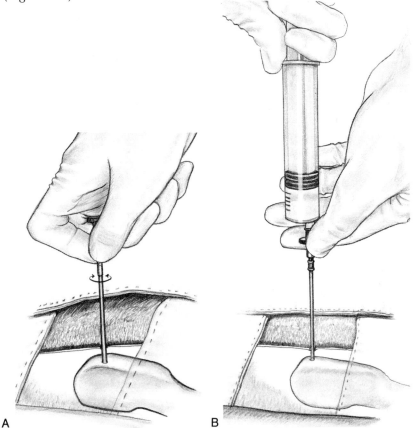

A   B

Figure 29-4 Aspiration technique: (*A*) Advance aspiration needle by applying alternating/rotating motion and steady pressure. (*B*) Aspirate marrow sample.

Technical Action

c. Aspirate small volume of blood and bone marrow.

8. Biopsy technique
   a. When needle and stylet are firmly embedded in bone, remove stylet.
   b. Advance needle 1 cm to 2 cm by gentle rotation and steady pressure (Fig. 29-5A).
   c. Loosen biopsy sample by alternate rotation and wobbling of needle (Fig. 29-5B).
   d. Partially withdraw needle, then redirect very slightly and reintroduce it into bone. Repeat rotation and wobbling of needle.
   e. Remove needle from bone by rotation and steady traction.
   f. Remove biopsy sample from needle using the expeller, and place it in appropriate fixative (Fig. 29-5C).
9. Apply pressure to puncture site until bleeding ceases.

Rationale/Amplification

c. Bone marrow usually is dark red, more viscous than blood, and contains fat particles. Less than 1 ml should be aspirated to avoid excessive dilution of the sample with blood.

8.
   a. The needle should stand in place after the stylet is removed.
   b. A comfort knob makes this step easier.

   c. Do not bend the needle!

   d. This repositioning obtains a larger sample and ensures that the specimen is severed from the bone.

   f. Zenker's fixative or formalin are used most frequently.

9. If thrombocytopenia is present, pressure should be applied for 3 to 5 minutes.

Trochanteric Fossa (preferred for cats and small dogs) Aspiration and Biopsy

Procedure

Technical Action

Performance Phase

1. Locate trochanteric fossa by palpation of greater trochanter (See Fig. 29-3B).

Rationale/Amplification

1. The fossa is medial and slightly distal to the point of the greater trochanter.

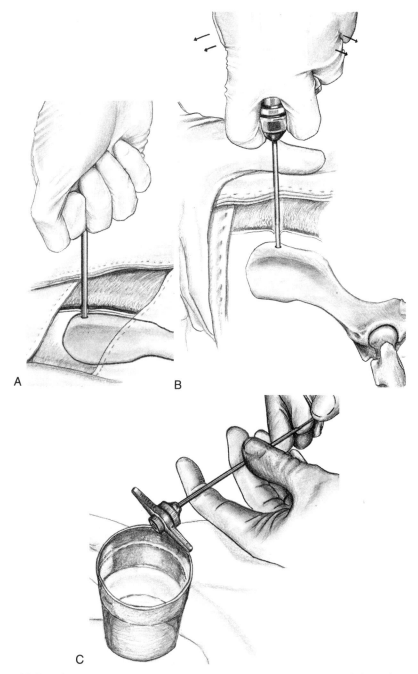

Figure 29-5   Biopsy technique: (*A*) Advance biopsy needle by applying alternating/ rotating motion and steady pressure. (*B*) Cut off biopsy sample by alternate, vigorous rotation and gentle wobbling. (*C*) Remove biopsy by retrograde passage of expeller.

Technical Action

2. Identify trochanteric fossa and mark.

Rationale/Amplification

2. Orientation is facilitated by cradling the cranial thigh in the palm and extending the thumb along the lateral aspect of the femur. This allows manipulation and restraint of the leg (Fig. 29-6).

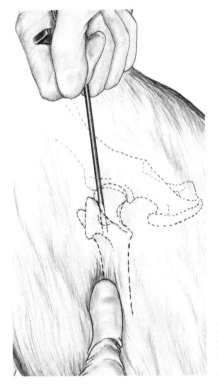

Figure 29-6 Restraint of leg and position of needle for trochanteric fossa bone marrow aspiration or biopsy.

3. As for iliac crest
4. As for iliac crest
5. Advance bone marrow needle, with stylet in place, through skin and subcutaneous tissue and into trochanteric fossa (Fig. 29-6).

3. As for iliac crest.
4. As for iliac crest.
5. The needle is directed medial to and parallel with the operator's thumb as it lies over the length of the femur.

Technical Action	Rationale/Amplification
6–9. As for iliac crest	**6–9.** As for iliac crest

NOTE: *A technique for aspiration or biopsy of the humeral head is not shown. The humerus is a good location (see Fig. 29-3C) for obtaining samples in anesthetized animals, but the procedure is more difficult to perform safely in the unanesthetized animal. Preparation and performance phases are similar to those shown for the other two sites.*

Bibliography

Perman V, Osborne CA, Stevens JB: Bone marrow biopsy. Vet Clin North Am 4:293–310, 1974

Schalm OW, Switzer JA: Bone marrow aspiration in the cat. Feline Practice 1:56–62, 1972

Chapter 30

CEREBROSPINAL FLUID COLLECTION

Good intent does not always result in beneficial outcome.

CARL OSBORNE

Collection and analysis of cerebrospinal fluid (CSF) is the most consistently reliable diagnostic procedure for diseases involving the central nervous system.

Purposes

1. To determine CSF pressure
2. To obtain CSF for chemical, cytologic, and microbiologic analysis

Specific Indications

1. Focal, multifocal, and diffuse dysfunction of the cerebrum, cerebellum, or brain stem, including
   - Motor deficits
   - Sensory deficits
   - Visual deficits
   - Cranial nerve deficits
   - Altered state of consciousness and mentation (*e.g.,* dementia or personality and behavior changes)
   - Epileptic seizures
2. Myelopathy, resulting in motor or sensory deficits

Contraindications

1. Congenital abnormalities, involving malformations of the foramen magnum, or suspected neural malformations in the region of the cisterna magna

2. Fractures, dislocations, or subluxations of the occipital region of the skull or rostral cervical region, resulting in severe distortion of the brain stem, medulla, or cervical cord
3. Suspected or anticipated brain herniation
4. Infection of soft tissues overlying the puncture site

Complications

1. No CSF obtained
2. Contamination of the CSF with blood
3. Herniation of the brain
4. Pithing of the medulla or rostral cervical spinal cord
5. Infection of the central nervous sytem
6. Respiratory or cardiac arrest
7. Vestibular dysfunction
8. Paresis/paralysis

> NOTE: *Serious complications may result when one is performing a cerebrospinal fluid collection, but problems are not common when proper technique is used and specific contraindications are considered.*

Equipment

- Sterile spinal needles
- Sand bags
- Spinal manometer (with three-way stopcock)
- Sterile syringes (preferably glass)
- Sterile tubes
- Sterile drape and gloves

Restraint and Positioning

Collection of CSF is always performed with the animal under general anesthesia. The animal is positioned carefully in sternal or lateral recumbency. Sandbags should be used, when necessary, to ensure symmetrical posture. The lateral position is preferred because it permits attachment of a manometer for measurement of CSF pressure and because it permits collection of fluid without the use of a syringe.

Cisternal puncture is facilitated by ventral flexion of the neck, which increases the dorsal exposure of the foramen magnum. Care must be taken to avoid kinking the endotracheal tube. The ears are pulled toward the commissures of the lips (Fig. 30-1).

Lumbar puncture is facilitated by drawing the hind legs forward so that the stifles are adjacent to the animal's umbilicus (Fig. 30-2).

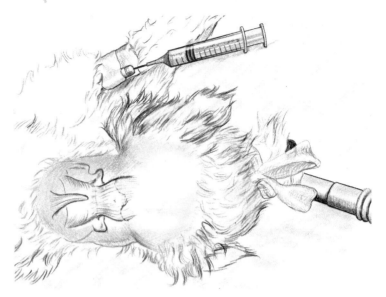

Figure 30-1 Correct positioning of dog for cisternal puncture.

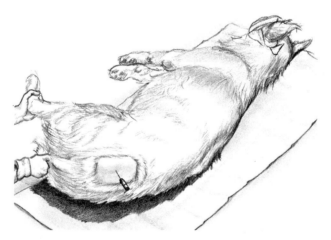

Figure 30-2 Correct positioning of dog for lumbar puncture.

Collection Sites

Cisternal puncture—In most cases, CSF is collected by entering the subarachnoid space at the cisterna magna. This site is particularly useful for suspected lesions of the brain. Anatomic landmarks include the external occipital protuberance, the cranial borders of the wings of the atlas, and the dorsal cervical musculature.

When the animal's neck is flexed, a slight depression can be seen or palpated. This depression is the site for needle insertion (Fig. 30-1).

Lumbar puncture—Collection of CSF from the lumbar region is performed less often in small animal practice because the subarachnoid space is narrow. Only small amounts of CSF can be obtained, and it usually is impossible to obtain a reliable pressure measurement. Lumbar puncture and CSF analysis ordinarily are performed before myelography, usually for evaluation of suspected lesions of the caudal cervical and thoracolumbar segments of the spinal cord. Anatomic landmarks include the dorsal processes of the lumbar vertebrae, the iliac crests, and dorsal lumbar muscles (Fig. 30-2).

Procedure

Technical Action

Cisternal Puncture

1. Clip hair from dorsal occipital and cranial cervical regions; prepare skin in a routine manner. Place sterile drape around site.

2. *Assistant:* Flex neck and pull ears cranially.

3. *Operator:* Direct needle with stylet in place through the skin and underlying tissue, toward opening between occiput and atlas (Fig. 30-1).

4. Advance needle with moderate force through meninges (dura mater and closely adherent arachnoid membrane).

5. Remove stylet and attach three-way stopcock and manometer (Fig. 30-3).

Rationale/Amplification

1. See Chap. 16, pp. 141–142. Attention to asepsis is important in avoiding microbial contamination of the CSF.

2. A depression usually is visible when the skin is pulled taut in this manner.

3. The distance from skin to cisterna magna is variable but is usually between 1 and 4 cm. The needle will often contact the dorsal lamina of the atlas. When this occurs, the needle should be redirected cranially in several small steps until it does not contact bone.

4. Entry into the subarachnoid space is sensed by a sudden slight loss of tension against the needle. With practice, this sensation can be readily felt in most cases. The animal usually will jerk or twitch if the parenchyma of the brain or spinal cord is penetrated.

5. Be sure the three-way stopcock is positioned so that the fluid may flow up the manometer column. The graduated column

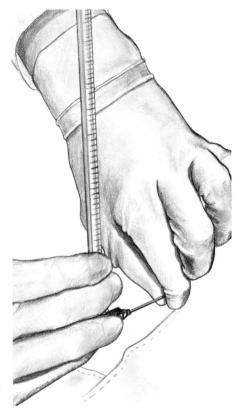

Figure 30-3 Attaching three-way stop-cock and manometer for determination of CSF pressure.

Technical Action

6. After pressure is measured, detach manometer and allow CSF to drip into sterile tubes (Fig. 30-4).
7. If very little fluid is obtained, attach glass syringe to needle and aspirate fluid gently.
8. Replace stylet and remove needle by steady traction.

Rationale/Amplification

should be held vertically. When the fluid stops its ascent, the pressure is read at the meniscus.
6. A small amount (0.25 ml) is collected for culture, and a larger amount (1 to 5 ml) is obtained for fluid analysis.
7. Collect as much CSF as possible to permit chemical and cytologic evaluation.

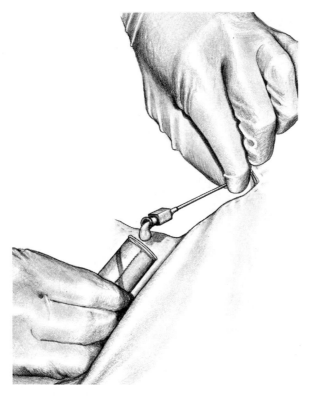

Figure 30-4 Collecting CSF by gravity flow.

Technical Action

9. Relax neck and observe animal for normal respiration.

Lumbar Puncture

1. Clip hair over dorsal lumbo-sacral region and prepare skin in routine manner. Place sterile drape around site.

2. *Assistant:* Draw hind legs forward.

Rationale/Amplification

9. When the procedure is properly performed, complications are rare, but the animal should be observed carefully for the next 24 hours.

1. See Chap. 16, pp. 141–142.

2. This position tends to open the spaces between the dorsal laminae of the lumbar vertebrae.

Technical Action

3. *Operator:* Direct needle, with stylet in place, ventrally and cranially through skin, subcutis, and musculature, toward dorsal lamina of the more caudal vertebra. An angle of 20 degrees from perpendicular to long axis of back usually is best. Keep needle in midsagittal plane by directing it parallel to dorsal processes (see Fig. 30-2).

4–8. As for cisternal puncture

Rationale/Amplification

3. Entry point is midway between the dorsal processes of fourth and fifth or fifth and sixth lumbar vertebrae. When bone is contacted (2 cm–8 cm below the skin), the needle is slightly redirected cranially or caudally until the dura mater is contacted.

4–8. During lumbar puncture the spinal cord is pithed, resulting in jerking movement of one or both hindlimbs. For this reason, the preferred puncture site is between the dorsal processes of the fifth and sixth lumbar vertebrae. If no CSF is obtained, however, remove the needle and reinsert it between the dorsal processes of the fourth and fifth lumbar vertebrae.

Bibliography

Kay WJ, Israel E, Prata RG: Cerebrospinal fluid. Vet Clin North Am 4:419–436, 1974

Chapter 31

RAPID EVALUATION OF BLEEDING AND CLOTTING DISORDERS

There is nothing so useless as doing efficiently that which should not be done at all.

PETER DRUCKER

Although many tests are available for evaluation of coagulation factors and platelets, the activated clotting time and bleeding time are inexpensive, easy, and require no sophisticated equipment or reagents. Each test can be performed in minutes at most veterinary facilities.

BLEEDING TIME

Bleeding time is a clinical evaluation of primary hemostasis. It is the time between the making of a small incision and the moment when bleeding ceases.

Purposes

1. To evaluate platelet function in animals with a normal platelet count
2. To screen animals with hemorrhagic diatheses for von Willebrand's disease

Specific Indications

1. Petechial or ecchymotic hemorrhages
2. Persistent epistaxis, hematuria, or hematochezia

Contraindications

1. Clinically evident prolonged bleeding (*e.g.,* at venipuncture sites)
2. Severe anemia
3. Severe thrombocytopenia

Complications

1. Prolonged bleeding
2. Infection of incision sites

Equipment Needed

- Tourniquet (pneumatic cuff or rubber strap and hemostatic forceps)
- Stopwatch with sweep second hand
- Filter paper (Whatman No. 1 discs)
- Skin preparation materials
    Povidone–iodine surgical scrub
    Sterile gauze sponges (2″ × 2″)
    70% alcohol
- Clipper with No. 40 blade
- Template and No. 11 scalpel blade (Fig. 31-1*A*)
    or
- Simplate-II bleeding time device* (Fig. 31-1*B*)
    or
- Commercial pet toenail clippers (guillotine or scissors type, Fig. 31-1*C*)

Restraint and Positioning

Little restraint is needed for most dogs and cats. The animal is held in sternal or lateral recumbency by an assistant.

*General Diagnostics, Division of Warner-Lambert Company, Morris Plains, NJ 07950.

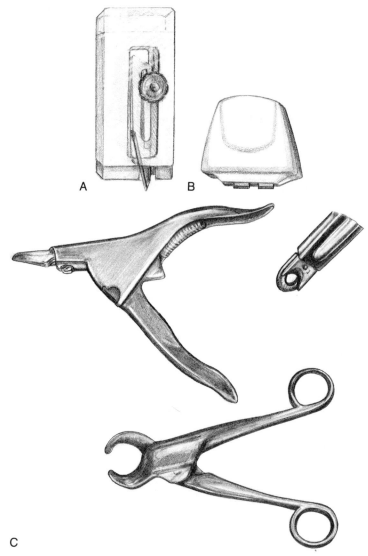

Figure 31-1 Equipment needed for obtaining template and cuticle bleeding time: (*A*) template and No. 11 scalpel blade, (*B*) Simplate-II bleeding time device, and (*C*) guillotine- and scissors-type pet toenail clippers.

Template Bleeding Time

Procedure

Technical Action

1. Carefully clip hair from 3-inch square area of skin on dorsolateral surface of midantebrachium.

2. Scrub clipped area of skin gently.

3. Apply tourniquet to leg above elbow. Wait 30 to 60 seconds before proceeding.

4. Make several incisions of uniform depth and length (Fig. 31-2).

Rationale/Amplification

1. Even a short-hair coat will prevent proper assessment of the cessation of bleeding. In addition, long hairs may provide an increased chance for wound contamination.

2. See Chap. 16, pp. 141–142. Careful clipping and scrubbing is essential to avoid skin irritation, which could result in surface capillary trauma and increased capillary perfusion.

3. The tourniquet helps to standardize capillary perfusion in the test leg.

4. Use either the Simplate-II bleeding time device* or a template (Fig. 31-2A) and No. 11 scalpel blade (Fig. 31-2B). Avoid placing the device directly over the cephalic vein.

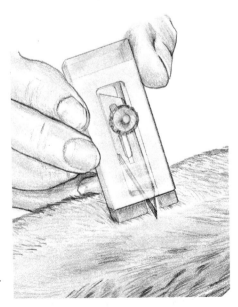

Figure 31-2 Making skin incisions with template and No. 11 scalpel blade.

*General Diagnostics, Division of Warner–Lambert Company, Morris Plains, NJ 07950.

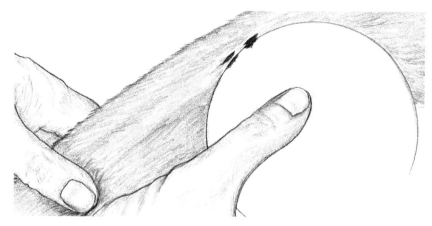

Figure 31-3 Blotting blood droplets with filter paper.

Technical Action

5. Remove incision device and start stopwatch.
6. After 30 seconds, blot the blood droplet that accumulates at incision sites with dry filter paper (Fig. 31-3).
7. Repeat blotting every 30 seconds until blood no longer stains the filter paper. Stop watch and record the total elapsed time.

8. Remove tourniquet and apply cotton ball or gauze bandage, as for venipuncture.

Rationale/Amplification

5. Do not separate incision edges or otherwise disturb the wounds.
6. Bring the filter paper close to the incisions without touching the wound edges.

7. Normal expected range is 4 to 5 minutes. If incisions bleed inequal lengths of time, use longest time obtained. Animals with bleeding disorders frequently bleed longer and more profusely.
8. See Chapter 2, p. 22, Nos. 11 to 12. If bleeding persists, consider placing a pressure bandage.

Cuticle Bleeding Time

Procedure

Technical Action

1. Wipe toenail and blades of toenail clipper with 70% alcohol. Allow to dry for at least 30 seconds.

Rationale/Amplification

1. Application of an antiseptic such as alcohol minimizes the possibility of infection of the nail.

Technical Action

2. Clip nail slightly too short to initiate bleeding (Fig. 31-4).

3. Allow the nail to bleed naturally.

4. Repeat Nos. 1 to 3 on a second nail to recheck results.

Rationale/Amplification

2. See Chap. 11, pp. 107–109. Darkly pigmented nails should be clipped in small (1-mm) increments until bleeding starts; in white nails, the nail matrix (blood supply) is visible so that an exact clip can be performed.

3. Do not squeeze foot, toes, or nails. Droplets of blood should not be blotted. Bleeding should stop normally within 2 to 5 minutes.

4. Bleeding may continue for 15 minutes or more in animals with von Willebrand's disease or other platelet disorders. Hemophiliacs will often stop bleeding after 2 to 3 minutes but will then restart and bleed indefinitely.

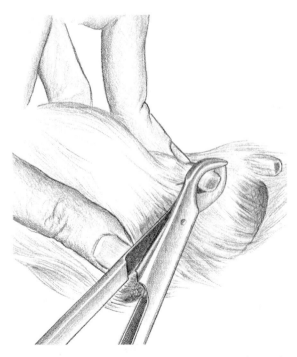

Figure 31-4 Clipping nail to level of blood vessels.

ACTIVATED CLOTTING TIME

Activated Clotting Time is a rapid test for evaluating the intrinsic and common coagulation pathways. It is the elapsed time between mixture of whole blood with a surface activator and the development of a fibrin clot.

Purposes

1. To aid in the diagnosis of specific coagulation disorders
2. To identify animals with subclinical coagulation disorders before the implementation of invasive or traumatic diagnostic procedures
3. To monitor serially anticoagulant therapy
4. To evaluate serially progression or regression of coagulopathies

Specific Indications

1. Spontaneous subcutaneous hematomas
2. Hemarthrosis
3. Suffusion hemorrhages
4. Prolonged postoperative bleeding

Equipment Needed

- Vacutainer† holder and needles
- Vacutainer clotting time test tubes containing activator, and standard clot tubes
- 37°C heating block or water bath
- Stopwatch with sweep second-hand

> NOTE: *When the procedure is performed in the field, warming the tube in a pocket or in the palm may be substituted for the heating block or bath.*

Restraint and Positioning

The animal is held in sternal recumbency, with forelegs extended forward and ventrally and the neck extended dorsally, as for routine jugular venipuncture (see Chap. 2).

Procedure

Technical Action	Rationale/Amplification
1. Preheat tubes in heating block or bath. Prepare skin and distend jugular vein as if for routine venipuncture.	1. See Chapter 2, pp. 19–20.

† Becton, Dickinson and Company, Rutherford, NJ 07070.

Technical Action

2. Puncture vein with one smooth stroke of sterile needle.

3. Insert standard clot tube in holder and push tube until needle punctures tube stopper. Collect 1 ml to 2 ml of blood.

4. Disconnect tube from holder while keeping needle within lumen of vein. Discard tube or save for serum tests.

5. Insert tube containing activator into holder and puncture stopper with needle.

6. Start stopwatch the instant blood enters the tube, and continue collection until blood stops flowing into the tube.

7. Immediately disconnect tube from holder, gently invert it three times and place tube in heating block or water bath.
Assistant: Apply digital pressure to venipuncture site for at least 1 minute.

8. When stopwatch reads 60 seconds, remove tube from heating block or bath and invert tube gently once (Fig. 31-5).

Rationale/Amplification

2. It is essential that the venipuncture be atraumatic to avoid the accumulation of tissue thromboplastin in or on the needle.

3. Hold Vacutainer collection assembly firmly throughout procedure to prevent migration of needle and laceration of vein.

4. This first collected sample is used to draw any thromboplastin out of the needle.

5. Blood normally will appear in vacuum tube immediately.

6. Collection normally should be completed within 10 to 12 seconds.

7. Inversion ensures adequate mixing of blood with the activator.

8. Observe for clot in tube as blood flows from end to end. If no clot is seen, replace tube in heat source.

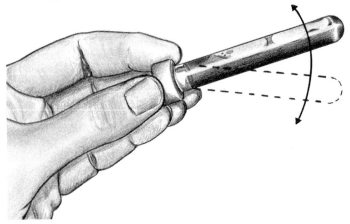

Figure 31-5 Inverting activated clotting time tube to observe for formation of clot.

Technical Action	Rationale/Amplification
9. Repeat inversion and replacement every 5 seconds until a clot is formed. Stop watch and record elapsed time.	**9.** Normal is 60 to 100 seconds in the dog.

Bibliography

Byars TD et al: Activated coagulation time (ACT) of whole blood in normal dogs. Am J Vet Res 37:1359–1361, 1976

Dodds WJ: Cuticle Bleeding Time, in Bleeding Disorders of Small Animals. Western States Veterinary Medical Association Annual Conference, Las Vegas, February, 1983

Middleton DJ, Watson ADJ: Activated coagulation times of whole blood in normal dogs with coagulopathies. J Small Anim Pract 19:417–422, 1978

Mielks CH: Use of template for bleeding time incisions. Blood 34:204–206, 1969

Remote from universal nature and living by complicated artifice, man in civilization surveys the creature through the glass of his knowledge and sees thereby a feather magnified and the whole image in distortion. We patronize them for their incompleteness, for their tragic fate in having taken form so far below ourselves. And therein we err and greatly err. For the animal shall not be measured by man.

In a world older and more complete than ours they move finished and complete, gifted with extensions of the senses we have lost or never attained, living by voices we shall never hear. They are not brethren; they are not underlings; they are other nations, caught with ourselves in the net of life and time, fellow prisoners of the splendor and travail of the earth.

HENRY BESTON

INDEX

Note: Page numbers in *italics* indicate illustrations; those followed by t indicate tables.